Health & Wellness

Insights For Vibrant Living

A. Calvin Ellison
2-26-12

Health
&
Wellness

Insights For Vibrant Living

Dr. Calvin Ellison, PhD

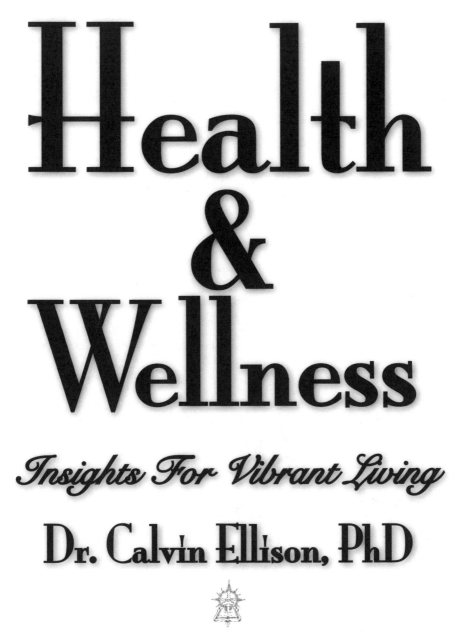

ARMOUR OF LIGHT
PUBLISHING
Charleston, South Carolina

Published in the United States of America by
Armour of Light Publishing
P.O. Box 21738
Charleston, South Carolina 29413

Visit us at: www.armouroflight.org

Design by Michael E. Evans

ISBN 0-9788590-0-6

Library of Congress Control Number XXXXXXXXXX

First Edition

All scriptures quoted from the Authorized King James Version unless otherwise noted.

10 9 8 7 6 5 4 3 2 1

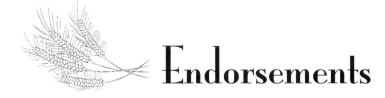

Endorsements

"I attended a workshop taught by Dr. Calvin Ellison, it was refreshing, educational and it gave me insight about the human body and what helps it to maintain strength. Dr. Ellison used the Word of God to show us how to take care of our organs and muscles. It certainly was and is information that will last you a lifetime!"

Pastor Tinnona Patterson
Words of Faith Deliverance Ministries, Inc.

"Dr. Calvin Ellison's nutritional and health seminar was a blessing to the Mount Zion Christian Church Family and me. Since attending this seminar, I have changed my food intake and have become very much health-minded. As a result, I have lost 23 pounds of unnecessary fat in nine weeks. I recommend the teachings of this book to everyone who reads it."

Apostle Donald Q. Fozard, Sr., Senior Pastor
Mount Zion Christian Church

"Dr. Calvin Ellison is an anointed man of God. I'm sure that every person who reads Health & Wellness Insights for Vibrant Living will find in it life-changing truths. I praise God for the ministry of Dr. Calvin Ellison."

Victor A. Marrow, President & CEO
Victor A. Marrow & Associates

"Dr Ellison's enthusiasm and ability to educate are only surpassed by his very sincere motives to bridge the gap between naturopathic and allopathic medicine. His lecture to our senior medical student class enlightened all our students on the study of Naturopathy. I was delighted to have him as one of the pioneers in alternative and complimentary medicine education at our medical school. It has been said, 'to teach is to shape the future.' Certainly Dr. Ellison's lecture helped shape the future of health care by his insightful discussion and living example of Naturopathy in modern living."

Julius Q. Mallette, M.D.
Senior Associate Dean for Academic Affairs
Brody School of Medicine, East Carolina University

"Our church was so blessed by the information shared with us during a recent seminar. Dr. Ellison enlightened us to some powerful truths concerning our proper nutrition, as well as the things we have been introduced to that hurt our health. We were so blessed and started to make changes right away. I recommend Dr. Ellison to anyone who is interested in a healthy lifestyle."

Apostle Ricky Pridgen
Covenant of Faith Church

"Just as it takes faith to be "healed", it takes faith to be "healthy." The believers who choose to take this faith walk with Dr. Ellison will discover the path to a healthier and more vibrant life. With increased awareness, a little self-discipline, support and faith, individuals, families and communities will be healthier! Through this training, believers will discover the power they have to break the family's history of poor health and promote wellness for future generations. Thank you, Dr. Ellison, for sharing the tools to prepare us for healthy living."

Barbara Pullen-Smith, MPH
Director of Office of Minority Health & Health Disparities

Endorsements

"Christianity points to the fact we should all approach life from a holistic perspective, by maintaining our spiritual and physical health. The scriptures remind us that it is important to keep our "temple" healthy. With this book, Dr. Ellison has outlined very practical approaches to a healthy life that can be beneficial to all age groups. His teachings, while based on sound science, are very practical. This information will help black communities promote health and prevent the devastation caused by health problems such as diabetes, cancer and heart disease. Dr. Ellison, through your leadership and commitment to service, the health of communities will be transformed!"

Pastor Ronald E. Avery
St. Matthew Baptist Church

"Having the opportunity to attend one of Dr. Ellison's Health & Wellness School Workshops, I found his teachings to be inspiring, thought-provoking and challenging. This book is a fascinating insight into the perceptions of a "mover and shaker" concerned about global health. It is an invaluable tool for understanding the holistic components for vibrant living."

Senator John Carr, North Carolina

"What a privilege it is that God has anointed and enlightened Dr. Ellison to tread upon kingdom waters and bring insights to the body that will ultimately alter the course of their lives. As a Pastor and Bishop in the Lord's church, as well as a Fitness Instructor, I believe that part of the deliverance of God's people lies in their mutual participation in destroying the yokes and bondages from off their shoulders by learning how to take charge of their bodies, which is the temple of the Holy Spirit. Let's take authority in the realm of the Spirit by taking dominion in what we eat and through the nurturing the body with natural essentials. Thank you, Dr. Ellison, for bringing this premium book to the Kingdom of God."

Dr. Haywood Parker, Senior Pastor
Truth Tabernacle Ministries

Health & Wellness

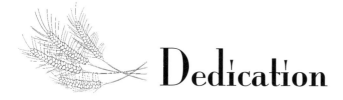

Dedication

To my Lord and Savior Jesus Christ who gave me the desire to learn about health and wellness and to share it with people around the globe.

To the Oasis of Hope Church family, a people who will rise to any occasion, challenge the challenges and strive to do greater things for the Kingdom.

To pastors and leaders who encourage the people they lead to better their quality of life through the knowledge of health and wellness.

To every individual determined to live a healthy life and be a model for others to pattern their lives after.

To my wife, Judy, whom I love with all my heart and who graciously follows me in the truths that are revealed to me.

Health & Wellness

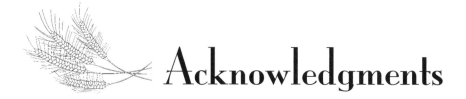

Acknowledgments

To Pastor Aaron Knight who uncompromisingly modeled a nutritional lifestyle before me that inspired me to change my diet.

To Traci Knight, thanks for working so willingly and enthusiastically to see this book through to completion. May God reward you a thousand times over.

To Dr. David Molapo, thank you for loving the people of South Africa so much that you would promote their total well-being: spirit, soul and body.

Health & Wellness

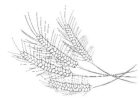# Table Of Contents

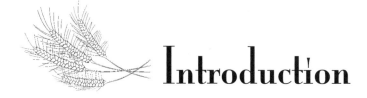

Introduction

You should live forever and never be sick. That was God's original plan for man. Sickness, disease, poverty and death were never intended to be in the vocabulary or experience of any human being. It was only after the fall of man that these enemies of God gained entrance into the human arena.

Before the fall of man, God had all ready laid the foundation for man's well being (spirit, soul, and body). For man's spirit to be nurtured, man was to stay in fellowship with God. For man's mind to be nurtured, he was to feed on God's thoughts only! There are so many psychological problems today that affect man's well being because we haven't done what Isaiah 26:3 declares, *"Thou wilt keep him in perfect peace, whose mind is stayed on thee: because he trusteth in thee."*

Mental health is crucial to man's well being. Solomon said, *"as a man thinketh in his heart, so is he"* (Proverbs 23:7). The highest level of mental health comes from keeping our minds on --thinking on (Philippians 4:6-8)-- what God says about a particular issue. We will discuss this more in a later chapter. Nurturing the physical body that is an extremely important factor in good health. It is also important to realize that in order to have the kind of health God intended, we must develop a focus and a foundation for each area-- spirit, soul (mind, will, and emotions), and body. We cannot afford to emphasize one area and neglect the others and still expect to have a wholesome sense of well being. There must be balance. Balance is a critical key to life. Although we will discuss all these areas of man's make-up, most of our focus in this book will be on the physical dimension of man. Why?

I personally feel that with all the churches in America and around the world, man's spiritual side is being adequately addressed. We have thousands of colleges and universities that work diligently to educate the mind for successful endeavors in life. Yes, I know that there are nutritional programs on television and nutritional centers around the world, but I still believe there is yet a great need to talk more about the physical side of man. After all, we are still seeing alarming numbers of people die of heart attacks, cancer, and many other devastating diseases. It should be a part of the mission of every believer in Christ to close any doorway to sickness or disease. The bible teaches us how to close those doorways by teaching us how to manage our health.

All relationships, organizations or establishments have a foundation that supports their stability and guides their progress. So it is concerning man's health that the right foundation is needed. We must consider what foundation we are building on--facts or assumptions, truth or lies. Man's wisdom or God's wisdom. Let's look at the bible's emphasis on the importance of building on a good foundation.

"Therefore whosoever heareth theses sayings of mine, and doeth them, I will liken him unto a wise man, which built his house upon a rock; And the rain descended, and the floods came, and the winds blew, and beat upon that house; and it fell not: for it was founded upon a rock; And everyone that heareth these sayings of mine, and doeth them not, shall be likened unto a foolish man, which built his house upon the sand; And the rain descended, and the floods came, and the winds blew, and beat upon that house, and it fell: and great was the fall of it" (Matthew 7:24-27).

From this passage of scripture we can see that if the foundation is right, then we can have stability, progression, and success for years and years. King David asked the question, *"If the foundations be destroyed, what can the righteous do"* (Psalm 11:3)?

It is the purpose of this book to help you have good health success from a holistic, biblical viewpoint. It is chocked full of ideas, information, and illustrations. There are charts and lists, a bibliography and an index. There is even a section for you to keep a journal so so that these dynamic principles can become a practical part of your personal health plan.

John Mark said that he wished *"above all things that thou mayest prosper and be in health, even as thy soul prospereth"* (3 John 2). Once you have been born again, there is only one way to continually cause your soul to prosper -- that is through the renewing of your mind by the word of God. Who has more understanding about the body and its functions than he who created it, God himself?

Further scripture gives more faith in God's foundation. Paul the apostle said, *"Nevertheless the foundation of God standeth sure"* (2 Timothy 2:19). God's foundation is his word, which is his wisdom. Solomon declares in the book of Proverbs that God has made all things by his wisdom. In order to have maximum health, we must consult with the wisdom of God.

"Through wisdom is an house builded;" Solomon taught, *"and by understanding it is established: And by knowledge shall the chambers be filled with all precious and pleasant riches"* (Proverbs 24:3-4).

Your body is the temple of the Holy Spirit. It is the house that your soul and spirit live in on earth. I want it to be filled with all the health and wellness that you need to enjoy an abundant, vibrant life.

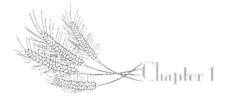

Walking with God and Vibrant Health

Because most of this book will deal with the physical dimensions of man and his health, the spirit and mental dimensions will be addressed first. Man was created to live forever in fellowship with God. In God's presence there is no sickness or disease. Physical ailments did not attach themselves to man until the spiritual cancer called sin came into the picture. Thus, we have the separation of man from God due to man's sin. The bible teaches that God hungers to share his love with us. In the Garden of Eden, God walked and talked with Adam and Eve in the cool of the day. That is what God wants to do with each of us, also. He yearns to be able to share his love with us and have us share our hearts with him on a daily basis. As our Creator and Sustainer, he knows what we need even more than we do, and he answers our questions even before we ask.

God's heart was broken when sin entered into Adam and Eve's lives and stole away the relationship he had with them. The tempter tempted Adam and Eve to live like gods themselves rather than enjoy the flow of God's life through them. In choosing to look to self, rather than looking beyond to the wonderful Giver of Life, Adam and Eve cut off much of the flow of God within them. In cutting off the flow of God's life, Adam and Eve began to walk outside the shield of God's divine countenance, thus exposing their physical as well as spiritual and mental dimension to the effects of sin. God's presence was to be a protective shield.

When sin entered man's spirit, his physical body became subjected to sickness and disease. You see, man was created to dwell in the environment of God's presence for security, provision, growth, and health. There is no sickness, disease or infirmity that can live in the realm of God's presence. It is important to know that all of man's physical problems originated from his spiritual problem, of being disconnected from God's presence.

When man was disconnected from God's presence, he, of course, lost access to the benefit of hearing the voice of God. I believe that there are some things we simply wouldn't do if we had a greater sensitivity to the voice of God (about our bodies) as Adam had before the fall. Many people have become so insensitive to God's voice (about proper health and nutrition) that when God does say something about health or eating right, they don't believe that it is God speaking. We must remember that God will speak to us about anything that we are open to. Ultimate destruction comes because we fail to heed the voice of God about a particular matter.

God has so orchestrated things that anyone (especially believers) can hear the voice of God. God's voice or what he speaks is found in his word--the bible. So when we read and meditate on the scriptures, we are actually hearing God's voice. If we act upon what God's word (or voice) says, then we will have health and happiness; if not we will have sickness and despair. As any good parent would do for his or her child, God is always giving us instruction for abundant living through his word. Note what Solomon (the wisest man who ever lived) said about the importance of hearing and responding to the instructions of God--

"Turn you at my reproof: behold, I will pour out my spirit into you, I will make known my words unto you. Because I have called, and ye refused; I have stretched out my hand, and no man regarded; But ye have set at nought all my counsel, and would know of my reproof: I also will laugh at your calamity; I will mock when your fear cometh; When your fear cometh as desolation, and your destruction cometh as a whirlwind; when distress and anguish cometh upon you. Then shall they call upon me, but I will not answer; they shall seek me early, but shall not find me: For that they hated knowledge, and did not choose the fear of the Lord: They would none of my counsel: they despised all of my reproof."

In terms of health, what Solomon said is even what believers in God do. They reject his counsel about health and plunge headlong into sicknesses and diseases. Wouldn't it be nice if God's children were the healthiest people in the world? Wouldn't it be nice if they were the most vivacious, active, spontaneous, and creative? Wouldn't it be nice if they lived the longest, accomplished the most, and became the most outstanding leaders the world has ever seen? Wouldn't it be nice if they didn't get the diseases common to the rest of the world because they knew how to live sanctified lives according to the word of God? God does not want to see anyone perishing, especially his children, but we must adhere to his counsel on health in order for sickness and disease not to be a part of our lives. We can reap rewards only in the areas where we have been obedient. So sow obedience to God's word in the area of health and nutrition and reap a healthy, stress-free body.

Much time has been lost, many families are disarrayed, and many lives destroyed because of trying to cure all of man's physical problems without considering whether spiritual laws are being violated or not. There are several spiritual principles I want to share with you (as a pastor) that I've seen over the years. I want to help restore health to individuals from a spiritual level. First there's the admonition of Solomon in Proverbs 4:20-22 (To guard our hearts by keeping God's word in it). *"My son, attend to my words; incline thine ear unto my sayings. Let them not depart from thine eyes; keep them in the midst of thine heart. For they are life unto those that find them, and health unto all their flesh. Keep thy heart with all diligence; for out of it are all the issues of life."*

It's imperative that we keep God's word in our hearts because the bible says in the above passage that God's word would be health to all of our flesh. This gives me reason enough to walk with God. You could say it's like this--walking with God promotes healthy living. Surely God, the author of life, isn't going to tell us to do something that contradicts healthy living. The above passage also warns us to keep (or guard) our hearts also because the forces of life flow from it. We must, therefore, keep our hearts from strife, bitterness, anger or anything that would cause the forces of life to be clogged up.

These negative forces will truly affect your health. Solomon further stated in Proverbs 14:30, *"A sound heart is the life of the flesh: but envy the rottenness of the bones."* Wow! That is powerful. This means that regardless of how I eat or exercise, if I allow the negative forces of envy, bitterness and strife to dwell in my heart, then they will cause destruction in my body.

The second spiritual principle is that of walking in forgiveness. Un-forgiveness or not forgiving someone of an offense will cause you to hold grudges, which after a time can cause tumors or ulcers. Many doctors are now tracing physical ailments back to grudges that have been harbored for years. I have learned over the years that all hurts have their roots in attachments. If we just let go of the experience, person or thing that distressed us at a certain season, then we can get on with healthy, vibrant living. Unforgiveness will zap the zest out of life and eventually bring one into a state of degeneration.

The third spiritual principle is that of *"keeping your mind on God."* The only thing that I can think of that would cause one not to want to think on God is sin. Why? Sin causes condemnation and shame. Therefore, one would tend to think of God as one's judge instead of justifier. The reason God sent his son to die for us was to bring us to the point of justification. Ask God to forgive you of sin and then move on and keep your mind on God as a loving father. The prophet Isaiah said, *"Thou wilt keep him in perfect peace, whose mind is stayed on thee: because he trusteth in thee"* (Isaiah 26:3).

The word peace means well being, wholeness (of spirit, mind, and body). This is important because our thoughts carry power. You become what you continually think on. We will talk more about thoughts in the next chapter. Concerning one's walk with God and how such a walk can influence one's health, Ed Bashaw in his book, Life Abundantly, encourages us to build a garden.

He said to plant and cultivate--

5 rows of P's – prayer, perseverance, promptness, preparedness, politeness.
5 rows of Squash – squash negatives, squash sarcasm, squash belittling, squash procrastination, squash mediocrity.
5 rows of Lettuce – let us be faithful, let us be positive, let us be cheerful, let us be giving and sharing, let us love and help one another.
5 rows of Turnips – turn up for church, turn up for meetings, turn up with a smile, turn up with new ideas and people, and turn up with a goal and determination.

You can see that the above spiritual garden will help promote good health and success in life. You may want to improve your relationship with God, or you may want to be sure that you will go to heaven when you die. Be assured that God hungers for a relationship with you and has expressed it in various scriptures throughout the bible. If you want a closer relationship with God and be a recipient of the abundant (rich, fulsome) life God sent Jesus to give, then pray aloud the following prayer:

G*od, I come to you in the name of your Son, the Lord Jesus Christ. I acknowledge that I have sinned and fallen short of your ways. I repent of my sin and ask the blood of Jesus Christ to cleanse me of all my sins. I receive this cleansing even now as you sweep over my soul. I confess with my mouth that Jesus Christ is the Son of God and the Lord of my life. I invite you, Jesus, to have first place in my heart and life. I believe God raised Jesus from the dead and that he is alive in my heart today. I forsake any evil ways and thoughts that I have harbored and this day turn my life over to Jesus.*

Health and Prosperous Thinking

"Beloved, I wish above all things that thou mayest prosper and be in health, even as thy soul prospereth" (3 John 2).

When it comes to vibrant living, the mind plays a major role in man's health. Apostle John in the above passage of scripture reveals to us that God wants above all things that we prosper and be in health. However, the key to prosperity and good health is what the latter end of the verse declares, *"Even as thy soul prospereth."* Therefore, it can be stated like this--you will prosper and be in health only to the degree that your soul prospers. To better understand what John is saying, let's get a clearer understanding of the words prosper and soul.

The word prosper means to become rich, be enriched or increase. The soul of man consists of his mind, or intellect, will, and emotions. It is impossible for the body to be in good health when the soul is ignorant of what it takes to have healthy living. Healthy living is the by-product of thoughts, concepts, and belief systems on or about healthy living. If you think apples are nutritional and will benefit your body, then apples will be a part of your diet. Please remember that the body gets its instructions from the mind. A sick mind will produce a sick body. A misinformed mind will produce a sick body.

Our mind works like a garden. We know that if we plant beans, then we will grow not corn but beans. We also know that if we plant one bean, then we will always reap more. If we plant a cup of beans, then we will get a bushel. The same holds true for the mind. If we continually plant the right thoughts about our health and nutrition, then we will surely reap a harvest of health. There is no great mystery to good health. Plant the right knowledge and, therefore, reap good, healthy living. Make no mistake about it--prosperity and good health are linked to prosperous thinking.

Now let us consider prosperous attitudes that will enhance your health. Prosperous thinking is victorious, harmonious, uplifted thinking. A prosperous thinker knows how to free himself of hostilities, resentments, criticisms, and irritated emotions. A prosperous thinker aims toward balanced, normal thinking which reflects his will to win.

Often it is mental depression and a feeling of defeat that cause ill health. Truly where there is a condition of ill health, there is a situation where the ill person has been subjected to internal discord of the mind, body or affairs. Prosperous thinking expressed as harmonious thinking helps to produce harmony in the body as well as in one's relationships and environment.

Bickering, quarreling or general confusion in one's daily atmosphere also affects the health of those involved. Teachers have often spotted this pattern in the lives of children who have come from disturbed, dysfunctional homes. The body is a very sensitive instrument, plastic to the thoughts, emotions, and words which are expressed through it and to it.

Had the ancient Babylonian sciences come down to us in tact, our civilization might be even more advanced than it is now. Not only did the Babylonians use strange stones of minerals for curing cancer, but they were also experts in the use of psychosomatics, various mental techniques even in hypnotism. It is believed that Abraham, who resided in the Babylonian city of Ur, learned of their treatment and brought it to the Jews, who effectively used it through the centuries. In any event, the writers of the bible seemed to understand that disease was caused by wrong thoughts and feelings. Their writings surely reflected that teaching.

All about us we see the need for transforming negative emotions if we wish to be healthy or to regain health. Cancer has often been referred to in recent times as a *"hate disease."* Those who contract it often carry their hate secretly so that the average person never suspects the emotional turmoil through which some cancer patients are passing.

If you are out of harmony with anyone, if you have been caused unhappiness in the past for which you are still holding a grudge, if you feel you have been unjustly treated in financial or private matters, if you feel that some loss has robbed you of the happiness that should have been yours by divine right, if you feel strongly about unhappy childhood and family experiences--then you may have every reason for your feelings and for continuing to nurse them. You may be able to justify those feelings in a thousand ways, but you mainly hurt yourself by doing so. Your health, prosperity, happiness, and peace of mind can and will be destroyed if you continue to harbor negative emotions.

Philosophers and wise men of all time have tried to point out that man's health is controlled by his attitudes toward himself and others. Hippocrates, the 4th century Greek physician, wrote, *"Men ought to know that from the brain, and from the brain only, arises our pleasures, laughters, and jests, as well as our sorrows, pains, griefs, and fears."* Plato declared, *"If the head and the body are to be well, you must begin by curing the soul."* The Psalmist David warned, *"Cease from anger, and forsake wrath; fret not thyself, it tendeth only to evil-doing"* (Psalm 37:8).

Solomon surely realized the power of thought and feeling on the body when he advised, *"A merry heart maketh a cheerful countenance; but by sorrow of the heart the spirit is broken"* (Proverbs 15:13). He went on to say, *"Pleasant words are as a honeycomb, sweet to the soul, and health to the bones"* (Proverbs 16:24). *"The light of the eyes rejoiceth the heart, and good tidings make the bones fat"* (Proverbs 15:30). Perhaps Solomon's best mental advice was this--*"A cheerful heart causeth good healing, but a broken spirit drieth up the bones"* (Proverbs 17:12). Truly a spirit that is broken, discouraged or depressed usually gets a physical reaction.

Developing a strong positive mental attitude is of utter importance if we are going to live a life full of vitality. Ed Bashaw gives us three keys in his book Life Abundantly that will help us develop a strong, positive mental attitude. Think success. Don't think failure. When you face a difficult situation, think, *"I'll win"* not *"I'll probably lose."* When opportunity appears, think, *"I can do it"* and never *"I can't."* Let the master thought, *"I will succeed,"* dominate your thinking process. Thinking success conditions your mind to create plans that produce success. Use success to help others.

1. Remind yourself daily that you will better yourself. Achievement does not require super intelligence, nor is there anything mystical about it. Successful people are just ordinary folks who have developed a positive attitude and belief in themselves and are willing to pay the price.

2. The achievement of your goals is determined by the size of your faith, belief, conviction, and commitment. We can confidently conclude that physical and mental health are inseparable, and, in the words of Solomon, *"As a man thinketh in his heart (mind), so is he (even in his physical arena)"* (Psalm 23:7 -- parentheses mine.)

Health & Wellness Nuggets

- The presence of God is the foundation for total well-being.

- When sin entered man's spirit, his physical body became subjected to sickness and disease.

- *"Thou wilt keep him in perfect peace, whose mind is stayed on thee: because he trusteth in thee."* Isaiah 26:3 (KJV)

- Physical problems are the result of a visitation of spiritual, mental, relational or physical laws.

- Unforgiveness zaps the zest out of life and leads to degeneration.

- *"Take fast hold of instruction; let her not go: keep her; for she is thy life."* Proverbs 4:13 (KJV)

- Walking with God produces healthy living: spiritually, mentally and physically.

- Prosperity and good health are connected to a positive thought life.

Health & Wellness

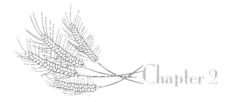

Chapter 2

The Original Diet

"And God said, Behold, I have given you every herb bearing seed, which is upon the face of all the earth, and every tree, in the which is the fruit of a tree yielding seed; to you it shall be for meat."
Genesis 1:29

There is nothing health-wise plaguing our society like the diet we are consuming. We are literally eating ourselves to death. As I began intently studying the subject of health and nutrition in 1994, it astounded me as to how far we (particularly Americans) had strayed from the original diet prescribed for man. On the path we are traveling, it's impossible for us to win the race for good health.

We are putting foods in our bodies that animals don't eat. We are dying of causes unheard of in the animal kingdom, yet we are the most intelligent of all of God's creations. People are taking better care of houses and cars than their own bodies.

As Christians, that definitely should not be so because the bible has declared that our bodies are now the dwelling place of Almighty God. If you'd ask the average Christian would he deliberately throw cans, paper, dirt, dead animals or any other defiling thing into a church building, he would reply, "Absolutely not." Why? Because we tend to respect the place where we are supposed to congregate to learn about God. On the other hand, we disrespect the actual house that God lives in--our bodies. Let's face reality--this is a form of insanity.

In the book of Genesis (the book of beginnings), God, the creator of the human body, prescribed the kind of foods we should be eating. Our problem is that we have rejected God's way to accept man's way (or our own way). Hosea the prophet declared, *"My people are destroyed for lack of knowledge; because thou has rejected knowledge"* (Hosea 4:6). The *"lack"* Hosea spoke of was not because knowledge was unavailable. The children of Israel didn't want to do what was right so they rejected God's knowledge.

We are allowing our taste buds to dictate to us what we should be eating or what we shouldn't be eating. Often times we go by the thought that if it smells really good then, we'll eat it, but if it doesn't, we'll leave it to the, so called, health freaks. Have you ever casually ridden by a restaurant and smelled the smell of broccoli or cauliflower cooking? What about cabbage? You probably haven't. Why? Because the foods that are best for you (although they do have a smell) don't impact the sense of smell in the same way the smell of barbecue or fried chicken does.

Fats have a *good* smell to them. In the Old Testament the fat of animals was to be burned before the Lord as incense. The Israelites could eat certain meats, but the fat of those meats belonged to God.

Eating fat will cause you to die prematurely today just as eating them would kill you in the time of the Old Testament. God has not changed his dietary laws.

We have rejected God's way and chosen our own. We have become what the Apostle Paul described in Romans 1:22, *"Professing themselves to be wise, they became fools."* We must honestly admit that this is exactly what is happening in America (the most technologically advanced nation in the world) and around the world. I am by no means trying to degrade our great country, but far to many Americans die of diseases that aren't even a major health-risk in some third world countries.

Eating injudiciously, unfortunately, is nothing new. The Prophet Daniel and his associates were placed in a challenging situation that caused them to have to choose between God's prescribed diet and the diet of the king of Babylon:

"And the king spake unto Ashpenaz the master of his eunuchs, that he should bring certain of the children of Israel, and of the king's seed and of the princes; Children in whom was no blemish, but well-favored, and skillful in all wisdom, and cunning in knowledge, and understanding science, and such as had ability in them to stand in the king's palace, and whom they might teach the learning and the tongue of the Chaldeans. And the king appointed them a daily provision of the king's meat, and of the wine which he drank: so nourishing them three years that at the end thereof they might stand before the king. Now among these were of the children of Judah, Daniel, Hananiah, Mishael, and Azariah: Unto who the prince of the eunuchs gave names: for he gave unto Daniel the name of Belteshazzar; and to Hananiah, of Shadrach; and to Mishael, of Meshach; and to Azariah, of Abednego. But Daniel purposed in his heart that

he would not defile himself with the portion of the king's meat, nor with the wine which he drank: therefore he requested of the prince of the eunuchs that he might not defile himself. Now God had brought Daniel into favour and tender love with the prince of the eunuchs. And the prince of the eunuchs said unto Daniel, I fear my lord the king who hath appointed your meat and your drink; for why should he see your faces worse liking than the children which are of your sort? then shall ye make me endanger my head to the king. Then said Daniel to Melzar whom the prince of the eunuchs had set over Daniel, Hananiah, Mishael, and Azariah, prove thy servants, I beseech thee, ten days: and let them give us pulse to eat, and water to drink. Then let our countenances be looked upon before thee, and the countenance of the children that eat of the portion of the king's meat: and as thou seest, deal with thy servants. So he consented to them in this matter, and proved them ten days. And at the end of ten days their countenances appeared fairer and fatter in flesh than all the children which did eat the portion of the king's meat" (Daniel 1:3-15).

Daniel understood the importance of eating God's foods rather than the deceptive foods of a ruler. Perhaps Daniel had read Solomon's warning-- *"When thou sittest to eat with a ruler, consider diligently what is before thee: And put a knife to thy throat, if thou be a man given to appetite. Be not desirous of his dainties: for they are deceitful meat. Labour not to be rich: cease from thine own wisdom. Wilt thou set thine eyes upon that which is not? for riches certainly make themselves wings; they fly away as an eagle toward heaven. Eat thou not the bread of him that hath an evil eye, neither desire thou his dainty meats: For as he thinketh in his heart, so is he: Eat and drink, saith he to thee; but his heart is not with thee. The morsel which thou hast eaten shalt thou vomit up, and lose thy sweet words"* (Proverbs 23:1-8).

Granted, Solomon's warning is more about deceit than diet, but Daniel knew that a vegetable, fruit, and grain diet was better than a meat diet--because that is what God told him to eat. Daniel proved that God's original diet would make one *"fairer, and fatter in flesh"* (Daniel 1:8-15), in other words, healthier, than a diet cooked in grease or synthetics. Even so, it must be proved again in our day that God's way--the natural, unadulterated way to eat--is the best way.

Let's examine why we must change from "The American Way" (since we are predominately dealing with our country) to God's way. What has happened in our country that is causing us to re-examine what is being served at restaurants, in our schools, and on our shelves in supermarkets? In my research I came across some information I felt you might want to take into consideration about our American Diet.

Dear reader, I submit to you that we can no longer live naively with what's happening in our country as far as nutrition is concerned. In light of the number of deaths from degenerative diseases, there are questions that must be answered.

John and Mary McDougall on the cover of their book, The McDougall Plan, ask several questions--

- **Are Americans among the most malnourished people in the world?**
- **Are the meat and dairy industries brainwashing us?**
- **Is the medical profession ignorant about our nutritional needs?**
- **Has our government given us faulty information on proper diet?**

These questions must be answered.

According to John McDougall (a medical doctor), the answer to all of the above questions is yes. Therefore, I see the need for more professional knowledge about the American diet.

Dr. Robert Garrison, Jr., M.A., R.PH and Elizabeth Somer, M.A., R.D. in their book, The Nutrition Desk Reference, give us some insightful information about the American diet. They say, *"The American diet is not as sacred as some might think. In fact the American diet has changed more radically and quickly since the beginning of the 20th century than at any other time in human history. In addition, the food supply of the 1990's mirrors the complex relationship between technology, economics, and social changes. By replacing manual labor with machines, industrialization has reduced the body's need for a high-calorie diet. New technologies have revamped the food supply by extending shelf-life, developing hundreds of new processed food products, and using flavor enhancers, colorings, preservatives, emulsifiers, stabilizers, surfactants, and a host of other laboratory-derived additives. The substances alter the taste, texture, color, feel, flavor, smell, and nutrient content of products lining supermarket shelves. The average store of the 1920's stocked 80 items. Today, a store with fewer than 10,000 items is said to carry a limited selection. This escalation in diversity has been bought at a high price."*

They go on to say, *"The nutritional quality of many convenient, prepared meals and snack foods bears little resemblance to that of the basic foodstuffs. These fabricated foods are ones which are processed more than necessary, i.e. doing more to it than we need to."* According to George Briggs, professor of nutrition at the University of California, Berkeley, *"processed foods might be fortified with some nutrients, but they usually ignore several trace minerals and fiber. Many are high in fat, salt, and sugar. Only half the calories consumed by the average American are derived from wholesome, minimally altered foods, e.g. vegetables and fruits, whole grains, extra-lean meats and legumes, and low-fat milk and milk products. The rest are derived from sugar, white flour, and fat. Life today is more affluent than at the beginning of the century. People eat out more often, snack frequently, and choose more convenience and pre-pared foods. Americans today are eating less than their ancestors and gaining more weight."*

What astounding facts. We can clearly see why we must challenge the conventional wisdom concerning the American diet with that of God's original diet. Unchallenged, this current American diet will continue to make producers rich at the expense of the American people's health and lives.

God gave the Genesis Diet or his Original Diet for long life and good health. This diet did not include meats. I'm not saying you can't eat meats--I still eat some meat myself. I'm simply drawing your attention to the fact that all of God's creature, fish, fowl, reptile, mammal, and man, were vegetarians until after the flood of Noah. (See Genesis 9:1-4)

There were no canned foods, additives or synthetics. The foods God prescribed for man took care of his physical and, to a great degree, his psychological well being. God's original diet didn't even in-clude the process of cooking. Adam and Eve didn't have a stove or microwave. The foods they ate were in their purest state – raw.

Now I know that the average person isn't going to eat everything raw--I don't. My appeal, nevertheless, is that we get as close as we can to rawness. It's better to eat steamed vegetables than vegetables cooked to the state of mushiness. Heat alters the chemical make up of foods and potentially destroys the nutritional value.

Why did God prescribe a specific diet for Adam and Eve? Why didn't he tell them, "Just go eat whatever you want to eat"? Is it that our diet is so important to our existence that God chose to bring the subject up? If you will take notice of the scriptures, you'll find out that right after God created man, he addressed the issue of what should be put into man's body. Now let's think about this a bit further.

Would you buy a new car and wait six months to return to the dealer to get your manual to find out what kind of oil is needed in it? No! You would want your manual the same day you purchased the car. You would want to know the requirements immediately so you would know how to properly maintain your vehicle. Otherwise you will not be able to get the most comfort, convenience, and mileage for what you are paying. So it must be for the greatest piece of machinery ever made--the human body.

You shouldn't wait until you are lying flat on your back in a hospital bed before learning what diet may have put you there! You and I need to find out beforehand. It may surprise you, but changing what we put in our mouths can stop most of our degenerative diseases. We must discipline ourselves to read labels, ask questions, slow down and simply observe more discreetly when we are in the supermarkets.

I like to watch people grocery shop. I often observe more people spend time in the meat section or down the isles of the canned foods section than over in the produce section. I used to do the same thing, but now most of my shopping is in the produce section. I love it. I now know that the produce section is closer to God's original intended diet. I'm not saying that everything in produce is A-OK, but it is more healthful than other sections of our supermarkets.

In God's original diet for man, the foods produced the nutrients that promoted the necessary functions of the human body. Animals, especially in the wild, don't seem to suffer from constipation as humans do. Why? I believe it's because they tend to eat foods that promote regular bowel movements. I've have never heard of an animal having to take a laxative Why? Once again, they instinctively tend to eat right and get the necessary amount of exercise that aids bowel movements.

According to God's original diet, starches, vegetables, fruits and nuts are the key categories. There were no meat or dairy products. Remember, meats did not come in the picture for men or animals until after the flood. Even then God gave guidelines as to how the meats were to be prepared and what meats were okay and which ones were not.

Consider the number of years man lived before the flood (on a vegetarian diet). Adam – 930 years, Seth – 912 years, Enosh – 905 years, Cainan – 910 years, Mahalalel – 850 years, just to name a few. After the flood (or when meats were permitted), man's life span went down to 120 years. For more knowledge on the meats permitted to be eaten, see Leviticus 11 and Deuteronomy 14. Also in these chapters observe that the word may is not a command to eat these meats, but meats were a choice.

Let's observe some more facts as to why meats were not prescribed in God's original diet (Excerpted from The McDougall Plan by John and Mary McDougall)--

1. Most of our teeth are flat for grinding grains and vegetables. They are not designed to tear apart raw meat.
2. Our hands are designed for gathering, not for ripping flesh apart.
3. Our intestine is long, like that of other herbivores, in order to allow for the time needed to digest nutrients found in plants.
4. Carnivores have a short intestinal track that rapidly digests flesh and excretes its remnants. Carnivores also have a great capacity to eliminate the large amounts of cholesterol consumed in their diet.

Wow! What important information for a generation that prides itself on how many meats are on its plate!

Dairy products were also excluded from God's original diet plan. In The McDougall Plan, John and Mary McDougall also present potent information on dairy products--

Dairy products have assumed a prominent position in the diets of affluent societies. The basic dairy product (whole cow's milk), is the food ideally designed for the nutritional needs of calves. This product is high in fat, protein, and cholesterol and low in carbohydrates. It contains no fiber. Products derived from whole milk include butter, cheese, cottage cheese, yogurt, buttermilk, skim milk, kefir, ice cream, whey, "imitation milk," and cow-milk-based infant formulas.

Because dairy products and meat have so many similarities in their macronutrients content, dairy foods can be thought of as "liquid meat." Dairy products are the leading cause of food allergies. They contain more than twenty-five different proteins that *"may"* induce allergic reactions in humans.

These reactions include the following:

•**Gastrointestinal** - canker sores, vomiting, colic, stomach cramps, abdominal distention, intestinal obstruction, bloody stools, colitis, malabsorption, loss of appetite, growth retardation, diarrhea, constipation, painful defecation, irritation of tongue, lips and mouth.
•**Respiratory** - nasal stuffiness, runny nose, otitis media (inner ear trouble), sinusitis, asthma, pulmonary infiltrates.
•**Skin** - rashes, atopic dermatitis, eczema, seborrhea, hives.
•**Behavioral** - irritability, restlessness, hyperactivity, headache, lethargy, fatigue, allergic-tension fatigue syndrome, muscle pain, mental depression, enuresis (bedwetting, often caused when the bladder tissues become swollen and insensitive to the feeling of fullness).
•**Blood** - abnormal blood clotting, iron deficiency anemia (dairy products are the cause of at least 50 percent of childhood iron deficiency anemia and an unknown percentage of anemia found in adults; this condition results from bleeding of the small intestine caused by dairy proteins and is not responsive to iron therapy until milk and other dairy products are eliminated), low-serum proteins, thrombocytopenia (low platelets), and eosinophilia (allergy-related blood cells).

Now let's observe the foods that were contained in God's original diet. First, starches are foods that contain adequate amounts of readily available calories in the form of starch molecules. Starch molecules are made of long chains of sugars, which are the basic units of our energy supply. Secondly, there are the vegetables. Research has shown that vegetables are the builders of cells. Vegetables provide valuable contributions of vitamins, minerals, fiber, water, essential fat, and protein. Thirdly, there is the fruit category. Fruits are the laxatives of the body and contain the necessary sugars that sponsor the energy the body needs. They also yield a generous supply of fiber and vitamins needed in the body. Then there are the nuts. Nuts as well as the other categories provide wide range of nutritional benefits from needed minerals to agents that promote health in the intestines such as that produced by black walnuts. As you shift from the American (Western) diet to God's original diet, you will be greatly reducing the amount of fat and cholesterol you take in and removing all animal protein.

Fasting for Health

"It is better to go to the house of mourning [fasting], *than to go to the house of feasting: for that* [feasting] *is the end of all men; and the living will lay it to his heart"* (Ecclesiastes 7:2).

Of the many biblical foundations for health, fasting is one that carries a cleansing and revitalizing effect on the body. Fasting is a process that has been used for centuries by people all over the globe. The bible reveals to us that fasting promotes health. Isaiah 58:6-8 declares, *"Is not this the fast that I have chosen? to loose the bands of wickedness, to undo the heavy burdens, and to let the oppressed go free, and that ye break every yoke? Is it not to deal thy bread to the hungry, and that thou bring the poor that are cast out to thy house? When thou seest the naked, that thou cover him; and that thou hide not thyself from thy own flesh? Then shall thy light break forth as the morning and thine health shall spring forth speedily."*

Abraham, Moses, Daniel, the first century church, and even Jesus, the Son of God, fasted. Jesus began His ministry with a forty-day fast in which he overcame temptation in the same three areas that caused man to fall. Notice that verse eight in Isaiah chapter 58 reveals that *"thine health shall spring forth speedily"* when you fast.

You see the body will heal itself if you give it the opportunity to do so. In order for the body to have good health, you need to--

1) detoxify your body
2) build your immune system, and
3) nourish your cells.

Fasting causes a detoxifying effect upon the body. Detoxification is the removing of toxic materials collected over the years from bad diet, poor health habits, and the environment. Symptoms of toxic overload include digestive problems, low energy, joint pains, headaches, depression, and mental confusion. When you are waxing a floor, you must strip the old wax before applying the new wax. Similarly, before anyone can expect to build or regain health, it is usually necessary to tear down and eliminate the old debris from the body first. Over a period of time, our bodies accumulate toxins around our internal organs, blood, and arteries. New life and energies will only come forth or as the Prophet Isaiah said, *"Spring forth,"* when we have allowed the tearing down process. Fasting is a tearing down process.

Unfortunately, we accumulate a lot of toxins such as artificial flavors and colorings, pesticides and various other chemicals through the foods that we introduce into our systems. These unnatural elements "weigh on" and cause degeneration in a system that was originally designed for natural elements only. The unnatural will only negatively affect normal operations of the body, thereby causing toxicity in various areas.

Many people are in dire need of a "good house cleaning." We have all heard the terms "spring cleaning" when we make a deliberate effort to carefully clean our homes of excessive dusts, debris or items

we no longer desire to keep. So it is with our bodies. We need to
have regular times of "spring cleaning" or fasting, which will help
new health to spring forth. Fasting is an excellent way to cleanse
your system, if done properly. Eliminating solid food and drinking fluids instead permits the body to muster all its resources for
"cleaning the house" instead of digesting foods. Fasting is truly an
opportunity for a new beginning, to recuperate, renew and regroup
lost energy and health.

Dr. Norman W. Walker in his book, Become Younger, declares:
*"Fasting is a very important part of any program related to the hu-
man body. It is very beneficial, provided that it is done intelligently
and not prolonged for a longer period than six or seven days at the
utmost, at any one time. The effect of fasting is two-fold. It gives the
digestive system and a great many of the body functions a more or
less complete rest, and at the same time it enables the body to burn
up and eliminate waste."*

Dr. Walker held a Doctor of Science degree in Health and taught
vibrant, healthy living for years until his death in the 1980's at 109
years of age. Dr. Walker further stated that: *"During a fast we eat
no food whatever. We drink large quantities of water or fruit juices
somewhat diluted with water. Such a fast usually has the effect of
stirring up a great deal of the waste matter, which has been allowed
to accumulate in the system. Some of it passes out of the system in
the regular course of evacuation and elimination. Much of it, however, is simply stirred up and lodged in some convenient niche or
recess, usually in the sacculations or folds of the colon. If allowed
to remain there overnight, we are apt to absorb some of the toxins
or poisons which this debris may produce. This would have the tendency to defeat some of the benefits we expect to derive from the fast
and may also cause some discomfort and excessive amount of gas."*

For a number of years I had back pains and excessive bloating from gas due to an overloaded, toxin filled colon. Upon coming into a greater knowledge about health care, I found that I needed to push away from the table more often and allow time for detoxification through fasting and other health-wise means.

In early 1996 I began taking herbal cleansing products and fasting several meals. I was startled to find out the amount of waste that was clogged in the intestines of my 165 pound, 5'7" frame. I observed myself having to defecate 12 times in two days. I knew then that I had to take my health more seriously than ever before. I was determined to find out what was involved in vibrant living and long life. Well, one of the major characteristics of people I read about who were living to be well over a hundred years old was that of having regular times of giving the body rest and rejuvenation through the process of fasting.

In a society that glorifies and worships, the food industry, I realized that there are life-producing benefits from the process of fasting. As I read Paul and Patricia Braggs' book Apple Cider Vinegar, I came across a list of benefits from the joy of fasting. Below are the benefits they listed that I believe will motivate you to want to skip some meals and allow a detoxification to take place in your body, also.

Benefits from the JOYS of Fasting

- Fasting is easier than any diet. Fasting is the quickest way to lose weight.
- Fasting is adaptable to a busy life. Fasting gives the body a physiological rest.
- Fasting is used successfully in the treatment of many physical illnesses.

- Fasting can yield weight losses up to 10 pounds or more in the first week.
- Fasting lowers and normalizes cholesterol and blood pressure levels.
- Fasting is a calming experience, often relieving tension and insomnia.
- Fasting improves dietary habits. Fasting increases eating pleasure.
- Fasting frequently induces feelings of euphoria, a natural high.
- Fasting is a rejuvenator, slowing the ageing process.

Health & Wellness Nuggets

- Fasting promotes health.

- Unnatural substances negatively affect the normal operations of the body.

- We are only as healthy as the diet we consume.

- People are dying of diseases unheard of among animals.

- People take better care of houses and cars than their bodies.

- *"My people are destroyed for a lack of knowledge"* (Hosea 4:6).

Chapter 3

You Are What You Eat (Or Didn't Eat)

Health practitioners have announced for years, *"You are what you eat."* To stop the plague of degenerative disease, we must judiciously consider what we are putting into our mouths. Many people never stop and think about what they are putting into their mouths. We give great consideration to the kind of gas or oil we put into our vehicles, but we don't think about the kinds of foods we put into our bodies. Well, just as your vehicle will run well when you put into it what the manufacturer designed, so will your body give you vibrant health when you feed it the proper nutrition.

Nutritious foods nurture the various cells, tissues, and organs of our body. A good rule to follow when considering what foods to eat is to eat the foods that match the chemical make up of your body. These foods can simply be classified as organic foods *(foods that man has not tampered with by adding chemicals, preservatives, or artificial ingredients)*. The bible talks about how the sins of the fathers can be passed down to the third and fourth generation. Well, habits and patterns can be passed down as well. If we don't exhibit nutritious eating habits before our children, then they are doomed to repeat the same eating habits in their generation, therefore, passing them on to their children.

In my family, we were not raised to eat nutritiously. There was no emphasis on what foods were nutritious and which ones were not. You just ate what was put before you, without questioning it. However, we as parents are responsible for what our children eat and will have to give an account to God as to what we are feeding them as well as ourselves. Problems that arise in our bodies, hospital visits, and simply a lack of vigor itself will cause us, sooner or later, to consider what we are eating.

Frankly, I think it is ridiculous for us to eat ourselves into bad health and then go to a doctor, pay him or her money to tell us to cut out the fat and eat more fiber--or you will degenerate into bad health.

In his book, The California Nutrition Book, Paul Saltman, Ph.D says, *"Food is fun, and sound nutrition need not diminish the pleasure."* More than anything else, it's the nonsense of nutrition-- unreasonable food fears and unnecessary prohibitions--that takes the joy out of eating. So no-nonsense nutrition is as much a matter of what you put into your head as what you put into your stomach. It starts with discarding food prejudices--preferring one thing over another simply because it's what your mother cooked even though you've now discovered that it's not healthy.

What nutrition can do for you depends very much on what it is not doing now. Remember, nutrition is the primary means of realizing your genetic potential. Without an adequate amount of nutrients, you are simply not going to live as long or as healthy as you could. Nor will you look as good or work as hard as you are genetically programmed to do. Neither will you be able to run as fast, resist infection, or overcome illnesses with ease.

We need to switch from the food consumption pattern that has become standard in the Western world--one high in fats and low in fiber--to one low in fats and high in fiber. This was not easy for me as our family was raised on greasy foods. We ate bacon and eggs, grits, biscuits and molasses *(with bacon grease poured on it)* for breakfast. Then for lunch we might have sausage sandwiches or pork chops and rice with green beans. When collards or cabbages *(awesome vegetables)* were cooked, they were cooked with grease standing on top of them when they were served. Even our home-made biscuits were cooked in a lot of lard. In other words, if grease was not involved in our cooking, then we didn't think our bodies would register – *"I'm full."*

Since those days I have learned a lot. Often I wonder how we even lived through years of nutritional ignorance. It was the grace of God that kept us alive. However, we can't keep eating like that and think that we will have a long life, full of energy. Fats will cause problems in your arteries and blood. The chemical make-up of the fat will rob your blood of its proper flow through the body as well as cause other physically debilitating effects. God, in his word, commands us to leave the fat alone. You are not eating nutritiously when you eat the fat.

Many of the foods on the market today have been stripped of their nutritional value. For example, white flour (which we seek to enrich with a few vitamins) has been stripped of its nutritional potency. We have been deceived into taking pride in the white items and leaving the brown or whole-wheat items alone. Beware of white bread. It works like glue in your intestines and also ferments like a wine in your bowels, thus offsetting the process of digestion. We must make the transition from white enriched breads over to natural whole grain breads that carry plenty of dietary fiber.

Again, my family used to pride itself on the loaves of white bread we had in our home because they were cheaper. We didn't even consider the fact that white bread had been bleached. When you bleach something, you change or alter its natural color and contents. Other white items to beware of are sugar and salt. White sugar has been found to be cancer causing. Research has shown that 24 teaspoons of sugar eaten in one day reduces the number of bacteria that our white blood cells will destroy by 92 percent. Also, white sugar has been found to have a drugging effect on the body. When it is consumed, it ferments, causing an acid to be produced that burns our cells. This causes a paralyzing effect on the nerves.

I'm not saying that your body doesn't need sugar. It does need sugar, but it doesn't need the kind that has been processed and stripped of nutritional benefits. There is a natural sugar found in fruits, vegetables, and honey. The natural sugars *(when consumed)* don't immediately jump into your blood stream, causing your blood sugar level to go up the way it does with processed sugars. The consumption of unnatural sugar will create pancreatic problems. Other problems that common sugar causes are diabetes, blood pressure problems, heart trouble, mental problems, and obesity, just to name a few.

Salt is another white item that we must beware of. Does the body have a need for salt? Yes, but only in trace amounts, and it must be in an organic form for the body to be able to utilize it. Salt in its organic form is called organic sodium, which occurs naturally in most all fruits and vegetables. Problems caused by salt are hardening of the arteries, arthritis, ulcers, distorted vision and blindness, high blood pressure tumors, and a multitude of other degenerative diseases. As you read the labels on most processed and manufactured foods, you will find salt and sugar in the contents. You must read the labels and avoid these killers. If not, over a period of time you will have consumed such an amount of these health-robbing substances that poor health will become obvious.

Eating nutritiously is key to promoting good health and long life. Therefore, let's consider other factors that are noteworthy in nutritional eating.

1. Eat meats that are low in fat content.
Chicken, turkey, and fish have been recommended by many doctors and nutritionists to be healthy meats. If you do fry food items that have skins, like chicken and fish, then don't eat the skins because they carry more fats in them. Baking or broiling is always preferred over frying. Health conscious people should avoid eating over five ounces of any meat in one day. Remember that meats stay in your body longer than fruits and vegetables.

2. Eat fruits and vegetables.
When eating or choosing fruits and vegetables, get the ones that are ripe and luscious. Items that are withering and rotten should be avoided. Fruits and vegetables should be thoroughly washed before eating due to the substantial amounts of chemicals being placed upon our crops today. Washing thin-skinned items in ivory soap will help wash away these chemicals that would poison your system. The closer we keep our foods to the state of rawness, the more nutritional value we will get out of them. Cooking foods to the point of being mushy grossly alters their chemical make up, destroying the enzymes and stripping the foods of their nutrients. It is nutritionally wise to avoid canned fruits and vegetables. They are infiltrated with additives and preservatives *(for longer shelf life)* and overcooked.

3. Beware of what you throw away.
Often we ignorantly throw away parts of our foods that carry much

of our nutrients. My family used to throw away the peelings of the apple, pear, and potato, to name a few. When it came to leafy items like cabbages, we threw away the outer, greener leaves and held on to the inner white leaves. Folks, the greener the better when it comes to certain foods.

Raw Foods verses Cooked Foods

We began this chapter with the saying, *"we are what we eat."* But to take this saying further, it is more accurate to say that *"we are what we digest and absorb."* The food cannot nourish us unless it is first prepared for absorption into the body. This is done by chemicals called enzymes, which digest the food and break down large particles into smaller units. In a single cell, there may be a thousand enzymes, each one promoting the union or division of substances. Enzymes are in all living things.

In their book Prescriptions for Nutritional Healing, second edition, James F. Balch, MD and Phyllis A. Balch, CNC, make the following comments about enzymes:

"In their primary role, enzymes are catalysts--substances that accelerate and precipitate hundreds of thousands of biochemical reactions in the body that control life's processes. If it were not for the catalytic action of enzymes, most of these reactions would take place far too slowly to sustain life. Enzymes assist in practically all bodily functions. Digestive enzymes break down food particles for storage in the liver or muscles. Respiratory enzymes facilitate the elimination of carbon dioxide from the lungs. Enzymes assist the kidneys, liver, lungs, colon and skin in removing waste and toxins from the body. Enzymes also utilize the nutrients ingested by the body to construct new muscle tissue, nerve cells, bone, skin, and glandular tissue.

Enzymes prompt the oxidation of glucose, which creates energy for the cells. Enzymes also protect the blood from dangerous waste materials by converting these substances to forms that are easily eliminated by the body."

We can see then that without the presence of enzymes in our foods, we can develop all sorts of physical problems, from the lack of energy and weight-gain to degenerative diseases. The late Dr. Edward Howell, a physician and pioneer in enzyme research, called enzymes the *"sparks of life."* You can't regenerate life and have vibrant living without enzymes, if they are the sparks of life.

Most physical problems come from ingesting foods that have no enzymes. I recognize that the truth hurts. It hurt me to realize that much of what I had been traditionally trained to put into my body was actually hurting my health. I am convinced that the more westernized we have become in the area of our eating, the further we have gotten away from foods that contain the *"sparks of life."* This is why our bodies are giving us a harvest of physical ailments. It's simply because we have been sowing the seeds of food stuffs void of what God intended for man.

Well then, you may be asking, *"what kinds of food contain these sparks of life?"* I'll tell you – RAW FOODS. Yes, raw foods, foods which most people don't get enough of. I know many of you reading this book may be asking *"how can you say we don't get enough raw food?"* I can confidently say it because it takes life to regenerate (reproduce, refresh or store) life. Remember the law of sowing and reaping. You reap what you sow. If we sow foods in our bodies that have all the elements that make up life, then we can reap life.

Raw foods (untampered with) will reproduce life. God (the Author of Life) would not have given us something that would produce degeneration and death. He actually never intended for man to die. Of course, when sin came into the picture, it brought forth or gave birth to death. Soon death will be totally done away with, but meanwhile let's not die prematurely by eating things void of life.

Food in its best state is raw. Never forget this. It is truth and you can't improve on it. If you have a sickness or disease, the quickest way to get rid of it is to turn to raw foods. This doesn't necessarily mean that every bite you take has to be raw food, but the more raw food you eat, the sooner you'll get well. Reality check, you won't hear this everywhere. For the most part, people would rather hear a lie or something that doesn't challenge the way they've been living, especially if what they were eating has been delightsome to the taste buds.

If you're looking for more energy, then exercise regularly and feed your body more raw foods. Again raw foods are full of enzymes and other life producing compounds that promote vibrant health. Even when it comes to weight loss, raw foods can help speed up the process. Foods will more readily be broken down and passed through the digestive tract when enzymes are present. So then digestion and elimination are more functional because of the enzymes in raw foods. The more regular we are in eliminating waste from the body, the greater our chances of losing fat and maintaining an ideal body weight. Don't misunderstand me. I'm not saying that all you can eat is raw food. I don't do that. But I do believe that raw foods need to be a high percentage of our daily food intake.

Much research has been done on a group of people who live in a remote valley of the Himalayas of eastern Pakistan. These are the

Hunzas. They are renowned for their robust energy and uncommon longevity. Their culture is not plagued with heart disease, cancer, diabetes, liver and kidney disease, arthritis, hypertension, colds, flu, tooth decay and many other diseases known to westernized societies.

In his book, The Healthy Hunzas, J.I. Rodale reported that *"colds are non-existent in Hunzas."* He said it was not unusual to see a Hunza male walking through snowdrifts in the coldest weather, bare-chested and barefoot. He observed one Hunza man travel sixty miles in a single day by foot in mountainous terrain, arriving back as if he had returned from a casual walk. Hunza women do not suffer menstrual pain or any of the other female complaints of our society. In Hunza, people typically died of old age in their sleep, without experiencing the chronic suffering that so often precedes death in our own society.

A combination of a nutritious diet (of which eighty percent is raw and fresh), toxin-free environment, sunshine, sleep, fresh air, exercise and a low-stress lifestyle have contributed to the Hunzas' physical well-being. You simply can't beat raw foods. They are the best when it comes to food. Why? Because that's the way food was originally given to us.

Eating cooked foods stresses the body, which must manufacture extra enzymes in order to digest food and compensate for enzymes lost in cooked foods. By eating cooked foods, you can actually lose more nutrients than you gain. Consuming sufficient enzymes is one reason that eating raw foods is so important. Cooked food contributes to our epidemic of chronic disease. Why? Because the cooked food no longer has the optimal nutrients originally manufactured in the food item. Processing and cooking foods is a cause of malnutrition, in addition to commercial farming and distribution techniques. The heat used in cooking foods damages nutrients and typically makes them more difficult to digest.

Consider oatmeal as an example. In the Food and Nutrition Encyclopedia, Aubrey Ensminger reports that dry oatmeal contains fourteen percent protein, but that figure drops to only two percent after it is cooked--a loss of eighty-five percent. The higher the heat and the longer the cooking time, the more nutrients your food loses. When cooking vegetables, steam them rather than cook them for an extended period of time. Remember that your aim is to nurture your body as well as to satisfy hunger.

Deceptive Foods

More than ever before, I am convinced that we need to conscientiously consider what we are putting into our mouths and feeding to our cells, organs and systems. Often we are ingesting items that appeal to the eyes, feel good to our touch and taste good to our taste buds. But do these items give us the nutrients that sustain optimum health, regenerate life or simply prevent sickness and disease? We really must ask ourselves, "what will the food items do for our well being?" I know some of you may say, *"Well, I don't have the time to be that technical about what I am eating, especially when I'm hungry and on the run."* But the truth of the matter is we can't afford not to be technical. We really need to raise the *"standard of seriousness"* about our health and stop leaving the responsibility to food industries, doctors and hospitals.

Years ago the Lord reminded me of what he said in His Word, that Satan is the *"god of this world"* (present age) and has spread his corruptive influence into every area of society.

"In whom the god of this world has blinded the minds of them which believe not, lest the light of the glorious gospel of Christ, who is the image of God, should shine unto them." (II Corinthians 4:4)

I was startled that God would tell me that the devil has people who are at work to manipulate our food supply. Of course to these people, it's all about money. Yes, money at the expense of our health and ultimately at the expense of our lives. We must train ourselves to be sensitive to what we eat. Now don't say you can't do it because we educate ourselves about what oil and gas to put into our cars and what we want or don't want in our homes. We simply must practice the thought that *"our number one wealth is our health."* Nothing matters to us or takes priority in our lives (other than getting well) when we are sick. Let's face it, most people get sick because of what they eat. God was so concerned about our well-being that He told us what to eat:

"And God said, behold I have given you every herb bearing seed, which is upon the face of all the earth, and every tree, which is the fruit of a tree yielding seed; to you it shall be for meat" (Genesis 1:29).

The problem is that we have gotten so far away from what God pre-scribed, that we are now deceived. Let me reiterate what I just said. The moment a person leaves what food was originally intended by God, he or she moves toward deception. Deceptive foods appear to be edible and sufficient for human consumption but in reality do more physical damage than good. Well, we know that God did not make anything that would destroy us because the bible declares that everything that God made was good. Paul wrote to Timothy that *"every creature of God is good, and nothing to be refused, if it be received with thanksgiving"* (Genesis 1:31 / 1 Timothy 4:4).

The problem is that our lust (which manifests as gluttony) for food has led us into deception. This is not a problem that began just in the last one hundred years. The bible reveals that even centuries ago, after the Israelites had come out of Egypt, they had this *"lust for food"* problem. While the Israelites were in the wilderness, God was feeding them with manna, a life-sustaining grain that God had provided for them. However they complained to Moses that they were hungry for meat. God gave them what they were craving, but afterwards they were struck with a plague.

"But while the meat was still between their teeth, before it was chewed" Moses wrote, *"...the Lord struck the people with a very great plague...they buried the people who had yielded to craving"* (Numbers 11:34-35).

Today's restaurants are attracting people not because of serving them whole grains, fruits and vegetables but because of the meats they serve. I often say that when you ride by a restaurant and the smell captivates you, it's not the smell of apples, cauliflower or brown rice. It's usually the aroma of fat coming from a particular piece of meat. Why? Because fat has a good smell to it. Under the Old Testament sacrifices, God told the Israelites not to eat the fat but to offer it unto Him as a sweet aroma.

So then food industries are making billions of dollars off of our cravings for things that God told us to stay away from. Gordon Tessler, PhD in his book, The Genesis Diet, makes some informative points on, what he calls, deceptive foods:

"Today the food processing industry makes billions of dollars a year trying to make foods better than the original. The spirit behind this deception is none other than Satan himself. Just as Eve was de-

ceived into believing that she could be as wise as God, man believes that he has the wisdom to improve upon the taste and appearance of the natural, wholesome foods that God created. Although processed foods may look good, taste good, and promise to 'build strong bodies twelve ways,' these foods are truly deceptive foods. They look like the real thing but they are not! Many of the foods we consume have imitation flavors and colors, and the nutritional value has been removed. These deceptive foods may fool your taste buds but they do not fulfill the nutritional needs of your body."

In actuality, we cannot improve upon God. The truth of the matter is, any food that does not match the chemical make-up of the human body will have an adverse effect on it. Altered food will throw off the body's chemistry, move the body from alkalinity to acidity and create an internal environment for the development of sickness and disease. Let's examine some of these *"deceptive foods."*

Synthetic Foods

Synthetic foods are foods made artificially by chemical synthesis. Synthesis means combining parts or elements to form a new product. What food companies do is tamper with originals (God-produced foods) and add something man-made to create something that stimulates our sight, taste, and touch. Please keep in mind that when something "new" comes on the market, it is the result of a strategy. The strategy is to get into your pocket book. It's all about money. It's not about your health and well-being, but money.

Can we trust foods that have been *"improved upon"* by the top chemists in our countries? The answer is no because God cannot be improved upon. We cannot tamper with natural things and end up with positive results physically. I believe we need to take the advice of a television commercial that played years ago that said, *"Don't fool with mother nature."* Synthetic foods are simply *"not natural."*

Artificial Foods

Artificial foods, like the synthetic foods, are not natural. They are foods made by human skill or labor. They are made as a substitute or imitation of the real. They appear real but are not real at all. These foods may not even have components of real food in them, whereas, synthetic foods may have some natural elements in them. Keep in mind that the artificial and the synthetic are often closely related. However, the artificial has nothing real in it. We've all heard of and seen artificial flowers. They are very attractive and at first glance look as if they are real, but they are not. They are pretentious. They aren't made of the *"real stuff."*

Foods Loaded with Preservatives

Foods loaded with preservatives are also deceptive in nature. They can have much of the real thing in them, but the major problem comes in what's been added to preserve them. These foods are loaded with additives. Much controversy has been associated with the potential threats and possible benefits of food additives. Additives serve to preserve foods for extended shelf life, to prolong a desired flavor or appearance, and to impact or enhance certain nutritional qualities to the food stuff.

We have a real problem here. You see, real food will spoil. After you cut an apple open, observe how it changes color after a short period of time. The same thing happens to other fruits and vegetables as well. God designed natural preservatives into our food supply to keep the food--but not forever. Real foods have life producing elements in them. All life under the sun is sustained by the law of regeneration, meaning that in order for that plant, animal or human to continue to live, it must continue to receive from God himself (or what He's provided for regeneration of life). You can't regenerate the cells of your body with foods that are artificial, synthetic or loaded with preservatives. And some additives and preservatives actually work against the regeneration process.

To further my case, remember the manna that God fed the Israelites with in the wilderness? Moses informed them to gather only the amount that would suffice their needs for a given amount of time. They didn't have to hoard it (or try to preserve or store it up) because the Lord would make sure they would continually have a sufficient supply as long as they were in the wilderness. However, some got greedy and took in more than what they needed, and it spoiled on them, just like God said it would. (See Exodus 16:16-21)

Enriched Foods

The term *"enrich"* is deceptive at best, and in many cases an outright lie. In fact most of us are often led to believe that the value of the original food has been completely restored through the enrichment process.

To enrich, according to the American Heritage Dictionary, means to make rich or richer, to make fuller or more meaningful, to add nutrients to, to add to the beauty or character of. Now come on. Let's think! Does what God made need to be made richer? Does what He made need to be made fuller or more meaningful for usage in the human body? I thought the Bible said that everything God made was *"very good"* (Genesis 1:31).

Does what God made need added nutrients? Does what God made need anything added to it that will enhance its beauty or character? Of course not. When we start tampering with natural things, we end up perverting them from their intended usage in the body. Remember, we cannot improve on what God has already done. God is perfect in everything He does. Food companies know they can make money off of us when they can make us feel we are getting more for our money. Have you noticed that God's wholesome foods are rarely advertised? If you never eat or drink anything advertised on television, you will probably never get sick and remain vibrantly healthy.

Let's not be fooled by advertisements. Deceptive advertisements are what captivated Eve in the Garden. Using the senses, Satan was able to sway Eve from what God had told her and her husband. Still the fall of man came through disobedience about what they were to eat. Don't let your taste buds lead you into physical bondage. Don't be fooled by what looks glamorous or enticing to the eye. Now let's review what the scriptures say about Satan's deceptive advertisement:

"Now the serpent was more subtle than any beast of the field which the LORD God had made. And he said unto the woman, Yea, hath God said, Ye shall not eat of every tree of the garden? And the woman said unto the serpent, We may eat of the fruit of the trees of the garden: But of the fruit of the tree which is in the midst of the garden, God hath said, Ye shall not eat of it, neither shall ye touch it, lest ye die. And the serpent said unto the woman, Ye shall not surely die: For God doth know that in the day ye eat thereof, then your eyes shall be opened, and ye shall be as gods, knowing good and evil. And when the woman saw that the tree was good for food, and that it was pleasant to the eyes, and a tree to be desired to make one

wise, she took of the fruit thereof, and did eat, and gave also unto her husband with her, and he did eat" (Genesis 3:1-6).

Notice, Satan didn't merely offer Eve something forbidden. He offered her something artificial. The fruit that he spoke of was not something God created, but something enriched. This piece of fruit was not just *"good for food,"* it was *"able to make one wise."* This fruit was not just pleasant to the eyes, it was able to open their eyes. In other words, Satan's advertisement had some *"hath God said"* in it. It caused Eve to question God's integrity, his genuine desire to provide all that they needed through the other vegetation that he had given them in the garden.

This is what caused Eve to go down the aisle to even consider buying the deceptive food offered. The word *"enriched"* is also what entices many people into buying foods with little or no nutritional value. We need to consider what we eat by the standard of God's Word and even some plain old common sense. Stop being fooled by advertisements. Read labels!

In his book, The Food Revolution, John Robbins gives us a breakdown of the percentage of nutrients lost when whole wheat flour is refined into white flour and supposedly enriched.

Protein:	25 percent
Fiber:	95 percent
Calcium, Ca:	56 percent
Iron, Fe:	84 percent
Phosphorus, P:	69 percent
Potassium, K:	74 percent
Zinc, Zn:	76 percent
Copper, Cu:	62 percent

Manganese, Mn:	82 percent
Selenium, Se:	52 percent
Thiamin (Vitamin B-1):	73 percent
Riboflavin (Vitamin B-2):	81 percent
Niacin (Vitamin B-3):	80 percent
Pantothenic Acid (Vitamin B-5):	56 percent
Vitamin B-6:	87 percent
Folate:	59 percent
Vitamin E:	95 percent

Of the 25 nutrients that are removed when whole wheat flour is milled into white flour, only five are chemically replaced (enriched). The only thing I have to say about the bleached wheat, dead bread we we grew up eating is that it is a wonder we are still alive to tell the tale.

I remind you, we can't improve on God. Carefully look at all the nutrients that have been lost to give us something that is supposed to be enriched or made richer. But we can't stop here. We must also think about what conditions such a food will cause in the body. Sadly, research has revealed that some of the diseases associated with white flour consumption are appendicitis, diverticular disease, hiatal hernias, heart disease, diabetes and obesity to name a few.

So why do companies go to the expense of *"enriching"* the wheat in the first place? The answer is simple, and simply stated in 1 Timothy 6:10. *"The love of money is the root of all evil."*

Our great grandparents kept a garden or lived on a farm. They grew their own food. They rotated their crops, like God told the children of Israel to do, so the land could rest and revitalize its nutrients and minerals. They ate raw fruits and vegetables while they worked in those gardens and they drank the pot liquor that boiled off of the foods they cooked. But promises of bigger crops that would grow faster and fertilizers and pesticides that would remove the added labor and "loss" of obediently allowing the land to rest soon deceivied them, like Eve, into eating that which would make them *"wise."*

Now our children have no idea where fruits and vegetables come from. They expect strawberries in the dead of winter, and turn their noses up at the dirt and drudgery of home grown vegetables. The big food companies have us. Because they have deceived us into believing that what they offer is better and easier, we have lost our ability and even our desire to grow our own food. If we want to eat, we have to buy theirs.

Processed Foods

Processed foods are foods that have gone through a series of actions and changes in order to bring the food to a desired state other than what God intended. Usually this is to extend shelf life or to make the food appealing to the eye or addictive to the taste buds. Of course, much of food's nutritional value is destroyed through processing. In order to make the food more appealing, substances are added during processing. Read your labels! You will be startled at the amounts of various substances that have been added to our foods to preserve them.

According to the 1982-1986 FDA Total Diet Study, frozen French fries contained 70 different pesticide residues. Frozen pizza had 67 industrial and pesticide residues. Frozen chocolate cake contained 61 toxic residues and milk chocolate had 93. Peanut butter had a mind boggling 183, including highly carcinogenic (cancer causing) aflatoxin, which is produced by a mold that grows on peanuts.

I warn you to take a second look at ingesting (especially on a regular basis) anything that's canned or packed. There were no canned or packed foods in the Garden of Eden. Adam and Eve ate only fresh foods that were not tampered with by man. Processed foods are not natural and cause all sorts of physical problems from weight gain to scores of degenerative diseases.

Genetically Modified Foods

These are foods that have been genetically modified with modern technology. The basic intent of food industries in producing these foods is to produce more food at a fast pace. Our ancestors did not eat genetically modified foods. I know that some will say we are living in a different time from our ancestors and that we are more technologically advanced than they were. That is true and I don't deny that. However, we must realize that the further away from the *"natural"* we get, the weaker our physical structures become, the weaker our immune system becomes and the faster we develop degenerative diseases.

I believe that genetically modified foods (GMF) are lower in nutrients, higher in toxins, and contribute to weight gain. Why? Because you can't improve on God and the moment we start tampering with what is already perfect for human consumption, then we create problems. Many of the foods in our supermarkets already contain genetically modified components. In his book, Never Be Sick Again, Raymond Francis unveils alarming information about the depth of genetically modified foods that are already in our food supply:

"Food industry journals estimate that about 70 percent of the foods in our supermarkets would test positive for genetically modified in-

gredients. *Most common are genetically engineered corn, soybeans, tomatoes, yellow crookneck squash, canola, papaya and Russet Burbank potatoes. Other foods are being developed, such as apples, rice, wheat, broccoli, cucumbers, carrots, melons and grapes; genetically modified versions of these foods are either in stores already or they soon will be."*

A 1999 study by Consumer Reports found that only one-third of U.S. shoppers realize that they are eating genetically modified foods. The FDA does not require these foods to be labeled *"genetically modified,"* and consumers do not realize what they are buying. People buy so-called *"fresh"* produce, unaware that these foods did not evolve through a natural process.

Wow! How devastating. We are being seduced into eating foods that chemically clash with our physical make-up and it's all about money.

Eating Moderately

Statistics reveal that over sixty percent of our population in America is overweight. One of the major contributors to a society plagued with too many pounds is overeating. When the Creator designed the human body, he designed it with laws that would govern the proportion of weight that each of its sections would have. Because we are breaking God's law of moderation, we are carrying unhealthy amounts of weights on body frames that were never intended to house it.

According to the American Heritage Dictionary, the word moderate means within reasonable limits, not excessive or extreme, mild. I believe that one of the biblical foundations for good health is eating moderately. Scriptures even warn us about overeating. Proverbs 23:21 warns: *"For the drunkard and the glutton shall come to poverty: and drowsiness shall clothe a man's rags."*

Go to the average restaurant and you will see multitudes of people with over-filled plates, especially at places where you can eat buffet style. If you tend to overeat, it is helpful to understand the physiology behind overeating. One of the reasons that we frequently overeat is that our bodies are not absorbing nutrients. Nutrients are absorbed through the intestines. The intestines have tiny villi or filaments through which the nutrients are absorbed. If these villi are clogged, then no matter how much we eat, our bodies are not nourished. These villi can easily be clogged by the waste products of foods that our bodies are unable to metabolize and utilize correctly. This is a good reason as to why we must be careful about what we eat. We may be clogging our systems. This clogging in a simple term is called constipation.

Dr. Norman W. Walker in his book, Colon Health: The Key to a Vibrant Life, notes, *"The expression constipation is derived from the Latin word constipus which translated means to press or crowd together, to pack, to cram. Consequently, to be constipated means that the packed accumulation of feces in the bowel makes its evacuation difficult. Constipation is the number one affliction underlying nearly every ailment; it can be imputed to be the initial, primary cause of nearly every disturbance of the human system."* When no nutrients are being absorbed as a result of clogging, the body sets off an alarm that it has not been fed, and even though we have just eaten, we want to eat more.

Another reason for overeating is the consumption of non-nutritious foods such as cereals, processed foods, and common junk foods such as candy bars, chips, and other devitalized products. So again our bodies set off an alarm declaring that they are hungry because they have been starving nutritionally. Until we give our bodies what they need nutritionally, the alarm will constantly buzz. Stuffing oneself will silence the alarm somewhat, but after a short period of time it will become louder.

When we have eaten nutritionally, the body should register a state of *"satisfaction."* A body that is malnourished cries out for food even when the individual is eating large quantities. When you sense the urge to overeat, instead of grabbing the junk foods, go and eat some raw fruits and vegetables, which are full of nutrients that will satisfy the craving.

Health & Wellness Nuggets

- You are what you eat.

- Many foods at the market today have been stripped of their nutritional value.

- Eating judiciously is a major key to good health and long life.

- Heat changes the chemical make up of a food item.

- Food in its best state is RAW food.

- Raw foods promote regular bowel movements.

- Our number one wealth is our health.

- Our gluttony has led us to deceptive foods.

- We cannot improve on the food God prescribed.

Chapter 4

Proper Bowel Movement

"For thou hast possessed my reins: thou hast covered me in my mother's womb. I will praise thee; for I am fearfully and wonderfully made: marvelous are thy works; and that my soul knoweth right well. My substance was not hid from thee, when I was made in secret, and curiously wrought in the lowest parts of the earth. Thine eyes did see my substance, yet being unperfect; and in thy book all my members were written, which in continuance were fashioned, when as yet there was none of them." (Psalm 139:13-16)

I have over the years read the above passage many times and really didn't take it seriously. I was *"spiritualizing"* this passage as well as others, failing to realize that we have our existence on three different planes: the spiritual, mental and physical. Of course each plane is necessary and must be emphasized. To be most effective in representing the kingdom of God, we must focus on developing each plane.

Well, like many believers, I was strongly focused on living right or walking in the righteousness that Jesus purchased. I was also focused on renewing my mind so I could stay saved and please the Lord with the new life He had given me. However, my body was beginning to suffer. I also noticed that many believers were also suffering in their bodies. Even today, when you see believers in a prayer line, the prayer request is usually about relationships, finances or their bodies.

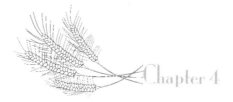

Why are so many Christians sick and even dying of diseases that our Lord paid the price to heal us from? Well, two things emerge in my mind: 1) lack of emphasis on the physical body from Leaders and 2) neglect. Let's examine these reasons carefully.

As leaders in the church, it is our responsibility to lead God's people into the paths that promote life (on every plane). Jesus said He came that we might have life and have it to the full (John 10:10). Understandably, not every apostle, prophet, evangelist, pastor or teacher has been called to be a nutritionist or fitness trainer, but we must allow those in "the camp" who have that assignment to lead the people in this area. People will not take to heart what is not being emphasized.

In light of the statistics revealing the scores of people dying prematurely from degenerative diseases, it's important that we in leadership become role models and or promote models of good health to the people. As the old slogan said, *"monkey see, monkey do"*; i.e. *"like priest, like people."*

The second reason so many believers are sick (and I realize there are reasons from the spiritual and mental planes) is because of simple neglect. Many feel that the physical side isn't that important. They feel that as long as they are *"deep"* spiritually, then every thing will be all right. They feel that they can just shout and pray away stomach problems caused by the bad foods they eat. Listen to me, my brother and sister. Your body needs attention. It is the house in which you live. Even your home needs, at the very least, periodic attention.

Look at what Solomon said in Proverbs 24:30-34:

"I went by the field of the slothful, and by the vineyard of the man void of understanding; And, lo, it was all grown over with thorns, and the nettles had covered the face thereof, and the stone wall thereof was broken down. Then I saw, and considered it well: I looked upon it, and received instruction. Yet a little sleep, a little slumber, a little folding of the hands to sleep: So shall thy poverty come as one that travelleth; and thy want as an armed man."

The man's vineyard in this story became overgrown because of neglect. To neglect something means to overlook, ignore, depreciate, pay no attention to, or to simply leave alone. That's what many people do with their bodies. They overlook, ignore and depreciate their bodies because they feel more spiritual dealing with their spiritual lives than with their bodies. They fail to realize that without a strong healthy body, they will lose some of their drive for spirituality. Then, as the slothful man's vineyard in Solomon's story, their bodies begin to deteriorate, age sooner and develop degenerative diseases. Every function and activity of your body's systems, day and night, is dependent on the attention you give it.

The food (both kind and quality) you put into your body is of vital importance to every phase of your existence. Good nutrition will regenerate and rebuild every cell and tissue that makes up your physical body. Your digestive processes and the body's ability to eliminate waste are dependent on the kind and quality of food you put into it. Few of us realize the damage that undigested foods and un-eliminated waste do to our well-being. I've personally had people tell me that they have bowel movements every other day or once or twice a week.

Not to have a bowel movement regularly (daily) is like having the garbage collector in your community go on strike for days, in hot weather. You and I know that the environment around our home will not smell good, especially if there is leftover meat in the garbage. Now I've been talking about the garbage being on the outside of your home. How much worse will be the smell of your home if the garbage was left on the inside?

I know this sounds gross, but it's time we look at the cold, hard facts. This is an extremely important issue. People are dying early all around us. The truth is that old age and degeneration begin in the colon. Proper bowel management will detoxify your body and help bring healing to it. If your immune system is strong, it will constantly wash all damaged and mutated cells and toxic poisons out of your system. But remember, your body can do a quality job only by the quality foods you give it. If you want an efficient elimination system, then you must give your body quality foods and exercise. You should not be carrying around Monday's meal on Thursday. You should discharge a meal within twenty-four hours after it has been eaten, not seventy-two or ninety-six hours afterwards.

What is Constipation?

For the body to continue carrying around the meals of previous days is clear evidence of constipation. The term constipation is derived from a Latin word meaning to pack, crowd together or cram. Simply stated, it means to have an accumulation of feces packed in the bowels that makes elimination extremely difficult. This is why many people moan and groan so--as if they were having a baby--when it's bowel moment time.

Bowel movements should be pleasurable. Your stools should flow smoothly and freely. Because of the type of diet we eat, many people have five to ten extra meals packed into their intestines.

With extra meals crowding the bowels, there should be no wonder why you feel bloated, tired and irritable. Who wouldn't? Then another problem arises when the bowels are stopped up or they are only partially functioning. Either condition will cause toxins to recirculate and be dumped into certain areas causing arthritis, headaches, abscesses and other unimaginable problems. Your best diets will do little good if the colon (the body's sewage system) is backed up. When the bowels fail, the whole body goes into a nutritional crisis.

The head doesn't get the nutrition it needs and we develop headaches, focusing problems and etc. When the joints don't get the nutrients they need, we develop arthritis, aches and pains and the like. Well, we could go on and on from organ to organ and from system to system. But I believe you get the point. We can no longer just live to eat, but we must eat to live. We must be discrete about what we put into our mouths. Constipation is actually our worst enemy. Many other ailments come out of a constipated colon (fatigue, asthma, colds, poor eyesight, hearing loss, nagging headaches and numerous other ailments).

What Causes Constipation?

Constipation is often caused by a diet high in fats, proteins, and refined products. In most households, meat is the main course of the meal. Many people have two or three types of meat at one meal. Thus their bodies are loaded with fats and proteins that slow down the movement of waste through the intestines. Then the problem is compounded when the meats God said don't eat are eaten. (Such meats are pork, shrimp, lobster, clams, catfish and others said to be unclean according to Leviticus Chapter 11.) By the nature of their make-up, meats travel slower through our digestive tract than fruits, vegetables, grains and nuts. Why? Because they are lacking in the dietary fiber needed to cause the bowels to flow freely. Then to compound the problem, many eat their meats with refined white flour products and refined sugar.

I can vividly remember the days when, along with family members, I ate a pork chop or ground beef sandwiched between two pieces of refined white flour bread with table salt, vinegar or hot sauce sprinkled on it. Actually I used to feel right proud bringing home the pork chops, pig ears, pig tails, ground beef (with a high fat content), three loaves of white bread for $1.19, three (2 liter) bottles of soda, two packs of cinnamon rolls (made of white flour of course) some fruit in a can and a vegetable or two that we eventually cooked to pieces. I can hardly believe we used to call that stuff a nutritious meal.

Of course in those days we had a lot of constipation, upset stomachs, gas, bloating, and other ailments. We thank God so much today for breaking through our nutritional ignorance and putting us on the path of a healthful life for the physical body. God is speaking to you right now. I know many of you are where my family and I used to be – eating the above and other un-nutritional products. Yet God is telling you to let go of the bad nutritional habits and come back home to His wisdom about proper nutrition that promotes vibrant living.

Another cause of constipation is the lack of exercise. Many people simply don't exercise enough. Exercise stimulates the lymphatic flow, which can help create normal peristalsis (movement) in the intestines.

Assisting the Colon

We must think of our colon as our friend and do all we can to assist it in doing its job for the body. The first thing to do is to chew your food well. Don't eat as though you are on a speedway. Your food isn't going anywhere. Take your time and chew it into an almost liquid form. Digestion doesn't start in your colon; it starts in your mouth. There are enzymes in your saliva that start the digestive process. Secondly, eat foods the body can utilize including lots of raw foods. Raw foods (fruits, vegetables and nuts) are full of fiber and enzymes that assist in the digestive processes. To deal with colon problems and even colon cancer, the American Cancer Association recommends that we eat four servings of fruit per day and five servings of vegetables. There is no substitute for raw foods in our diets. Raw food does more for our bodies than any other type. Too many cooked foods are directly related to a sluggish colon, intestinal problems, weight gain, indigestion and diarrhea.

The Power of Water

Thirdly, drinking plenty of water assists in proper bowel management. Countless studies have shown that few people are drinking water in any significant amount. The body loses ten glasses of water every day. The more dehydrated a person is, the more constipated he or she will be. I have talked with many people who say they drink water only occasionally and some who say, not at all. Some say they don't like the taste of water and they would rather have a soda instead.

These people fail to realize that they have trained themselves to want sodas over water. No child comes out of the womb asking for soda. The soda was introduced and then, because of the taste buds being tickled, the individual continues desiring something that isn't good for him. Water is so necessary for the human body. Your body is made up of 70 percent water. Look at some other water facts:

- Your muscles are about 75% water.
- Your brain is about 75% water
- Your blood is approximately 82% water.
- Your bones are approximately 25% water.

The consequence of not drinking enough water is that you won't have sufficient fluids in your tissues and therefore may become chronically dehydrated.

Dr. Leonard Smith, MD, Medical Advisor for Renew Life, The Digestive Care Company, said concerning Peristalsis/Hydration:

"To achieve 2 to 3 bowel movements per day, the peristaltic actions of the bowel must be regular and vigorous. Peristalsis is the natural wave like movement of the colon. This action, when functioning normally, moves food through the digestive system is less than 24 hours. There are many ways to stimulate peristalsis, but the most important way is through proper hydration of the colon. Most people don't know that constipation is often caused by dehydration. The key to hydrating the colon is to drink plenty of water, and if you like, you can jump start the peristaltic action of the sluggish colon by using hydrating minerals and gentle (non-laxative) herbs. Many "natural" products stimulate peristaltic action using herbal laxatives like cascara sagrada and senna. Cascara sagrada and senna are laxatives or purgative herbs. They work by irritating the colon, causing it to expel its contents. Hydrates of the colon are the key to making peristalsis occur naturally, and the use of ingested water and gentle minerals and herbs is a far better solution."

We just can't underestimate the value of water in bowel movements and any other bodily function. We will talk more about water in the next chapter.

A fourth way to assist our colon is through fiber. Fiber is found in many foods. Fiber works like a broom to sweep the walls of the colon from waste. Fiber helps to prevent colon cancer, constipation, hemorrhoids and obesity. Fiber helps to lower the blood cholesterol level and stabilize blood sugar levels. For years nutritionists have said, *"An apple a day will keep the doctor away."* Why? Because apples are loaded with fiber, water and other ingredients that help keep our bowels regular. Some other foods that carry lots of fiber are prunes, kiwis and pears. I named these because they are some of my favorites. Of course, these are all fruits. Remember your vegetables, nuts and beans have fiber as well. Back to the fruits. Fruits were designed by our Creator to work like laxatives in our bowels. I challenge anyone to periodically have just a fruit meal once during the day and reap the cleansing effect they have on the body.

Instead of depending on God's way (through what we eat and exercise), many people turn to laxatives. Why? Because we want a quick fix, especially after we've clogged the system with a lot of meats, white flour and dairy products. Laxatives have become "big" business. What wise businessman would not look at the health trends going on and not capitalize on our neglect in doing the right thing for our bodies. Of course, laxatives will eject waste from the bowels. This happens because the colon becomes so irritated in discharging the offending laxative that anything else that is loose goes out with it. The use of laxatives is not only habit forming but also destructive to the membrane of the intestines. Laxatives disturb the normal rhythm of the excretory organs. As a rule of thumb, under normal circumstances, it's always better to go natural in resolving physical ailments. If we will stick to eating what God prescribed (that which is natural), we won't have to turn to man-made chemicals to take care of a God-designed body.

Truly, God didn't put ingredients into the food to constipate us. So then, where are the constipation problems coming from? They are coming from foods that have been tampered with by human ingenuity: processed foods, chemical laden foods, genetically modified foods and foods that were classified as unclean for human consumption according to Leviticus chapter 11.

A fifth way to assist your colon in removing waste is to lubricate your colon with a good oil. I personally take flax seed oil daily, immediately after my meal. There are other good oils, like borage and fish oil, that are effective in providing us with a smooth and gentle elimination. In addition to the above ways whereby we can assist our colon, Dr. Leonard Smith, MD, gives some further recommendations:

1. Drink plenty of water.
2. Change your diet slowly, adding more fruits and vegetables. Supplement with a good daily fiber. Lower the amount of refined starches, sugar and processed foods in your diet.
3. Try taking digestive enzymes with your meals.
4. Exercise! If not daily, then at least three times per week for thirty minutes.
5. Lubricate your colon by taking essential fatty acids in oils such as flax, borage and fish.
6. When traveling, try to maintain a normal diet and regular sleep.
7. Create time to go to the bathroom in the morning, even if it means getting up a little earlier than usual.
8. Position yourself correctly when using the toilet. Keep the feet

raised on a telephone book or a device designed for proper elimination posture.

9. Do bi-annual cleanses using herbal combinations designed to support overall body and intestinal detoxification.

10. Use colon hydro-therapy hydration.

It's important for us to understand that improving digestion is the cornerstone to good health. When digestion improves, energy level improves, the skin becomes softer and cleaner, body odor reduces and the immune system is strengthened. If you have persistent, specific digestive difficulties, the best person to see is a nutritional consultant. Most digestive problems can be solved with relative ease, little expense, and no need for invasive tests or treatment. Remember, the best way to deal with any physical problems is the natural approach. Don't procrastinate. Be diligent about your physical well-being. After all, you only have one life to live.

Health & Wellness Nuggets

- It is the responsibility of leaders to be an example in health and wellness.

- Your bowels should be discharging a meal within 24 hours.

- Your colon is the sewage system of the body.

- Constipation is the result of a diet low in fiber.

- Constipation is caused by a diet high in fats, proteins and refined products.

- Digestion doesn't start in your colon; it starts in your mouth.

- Water plays a major role in regular bowel movements.

- Fiber works like a broom, sweeping the walls of the intestine.

Chapter 5

The Wonders Of Water

According to our Creator's design, water covers nearly three-fourths of the earth's surface. Then, as we look at the make-up of the human body, we also see three-fourths of it is water as well. I believe the Lord is telling us something of great importance – water is extremely necessary for life on this planet. Everything living--plants, animals, birds, insects, and of course humans--contains a certain amount of water. Nothing can live without water and nothing can be healthy without the designed amount of water remaining in its being. I personally feel that many people are taking the need for water very lightly.

There are many people who say they don't like water because it has no taste. They would rather have Gatorade, tea or soda. These people fail to realize that they acquired a taste for the Gatorade, tea or soda. Usually the desire for these types of liquids was developed because of the sugar factor or some man-made chemical that tickled their taste buds. You can train yourself to like anything if you'll keep using it long enough. However, water is a must. We cannot deviate from our Maker's design and expect to get the results he intended. Some of the aches and pains experienced in today's society can be solved by simply giving the body the needed amounts of water. People with joint pain and arthritis definitely need water to help provide lubrication for their joints.

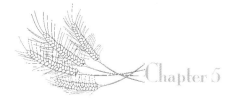

Water is the major constituent of all the fluids in the body: saliva, gastric juices, intestinal secretions, blood, etc. Now meditate for a moment. If water is in all the fluids of the body, think about how the body's organs and systems would function if given less water than they were designed by our Creator to have. They simply can't do their job at maximum proficiency when we haven't given them what they need. The continual deprivation of necessary resources leads to a breakdown.

Water is important for carrying nutrients to all cells of the body and for removing waste products from the body via the bloodstream and the excretory organs. This same pattern is used in our homes. We use water in our commodes to flush body waste out of the home and into the sewage system. If there is no water in the commode and in the pipelines, then the waste won't go anywhere. It will remain in the commode and cause problems in the home. This is what happens in the human body when it doesn't get the necessary amount of what it needs. We can therefore see where many of our physical problems stem from. Water is directly related to easing such problems as back pains, arthritis and headaches, and improving blood pressure.

Plenty of water promotes smooth, glowing skin. Superstar Tina Turner, who is aging beautifully, attributes her youthful appearance to drinking plenty of water everyday. The average size individual needs about three quarts of water daily. I know some readers are thinking, "I get a lot of that amount in sodas, teas, coffee and milk-shakes." Of course, there is water in these items, but we also need to be conscious of the fact that sodas are loaded with sugar and chemicals that impair our immune system. Teas and coffee (unless herbal) are loaded with toxins that rob the body of iron.

The Milk Question

Then there's the milk question--cow's milk, of course. I can hear some of you fussing at me at this point. What's wrong with cow's milk? First of all, it was intended for cows and not for humans. It is the most mucus-forming food in our food chain. From infancy to old age, it is a major cause of asthma, colds, the flu, sinus trouble, hay fever and tuberculosis. You should avoid dairy products and, when in need of something to replace cow's milk, consider almond or rice milk, soy milk or goat's milk. What? Goat's milk! Goat's milk is similar to human milk in it's nutritional composition and it is presented as an acceptable food source by King Solomon in Proverbs 27:27. Afraid you won't like it? Remember, you consumed cow's milk because it was introduced to you as a child and you habitually drank it until you got used to it.

Water and Liver Functioning

Water is also essential to proper liver functioning. The liver has the big responsibility of metabolizing stored fat into energy. When the body doesn't receive adequate water, the kidneys begin to malfunction and the liver has take up the slack. When this happens, less fat is metabolized. When less fat is burned, then more fat remains stored. So when the body does not receive the adequate amount of water needed, it's almost impossible to lose weight.

Water Loss

Replenishing the body with a sufficient amount of water daily is also important because of the loss of water on a daily basis. Often we are not conscious that we lose water daily. We do, in four ways:

- Through perspiration
- Through urine
- Through the lungs when we breathe out
- Through daily bowel movements

More water is needed in hot weather and when you exercise vigorously. During these times dehydration can quickly set in and lead to other problems. So remember to drink the amount needed, usually half of your body weight converted into ounces. In other words, if you weigh 160 pounds, you need 80 ounces of water per day.

By keeping in mind the following purposes of water, you should be motivated to treat your body right by giving it the needed amounts of water. Water maintains body temperature, aids in digestion, metabolizes fat and lubricates organs, cushions organs, transports nutrients and flushes out toxins.

Health & Wellness Nuggets

- Everything living contains a certain amount of water.
- Nothing can be optimally healthy without its designed amount of water.
- Water can't be replaced as a liquid by drinking Gatorade, tea or sodas.
- Water is a major constituent of all the fluids of the body.
- Plenty of water promotes smooth, glowing skin.
- Cow's milk was never intended for the human body. It was intended for calves.
- Water is essential for ridding the body of waste and relieving constipation.

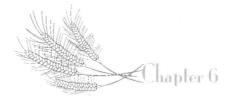
Natural Weight Control

"Know ye not that they which run in a race run all, but one receiveth the prize? So run, that ye may obtain. And every man that striveth for the mastery is temperate in all thing. Now they do it to obtain a corruptible crown; but we an incorruptible. I therefore so run, not as uncertainly; so fight I, not as one that beateth the air: But I keep under my body, and bring it into subjection: lest that by any means, when I have preached to others, I myself should be a castaway." I Corinthians 9:24-27

There is much concern about weight control in many nations today. Alarming numbers of adults are overweight, and the problem has spilled over into obesity (meaning there are health problems involved). Many people are turning to all sorts of diets, surgery and outright scams in order to get slim.

The weight crisis is not limited to any age group as we see even our children falling prey to this epidemic. Some people fight tenaciously to keep their weight under control while others just don't care. Then there are still others who are plainly confused about what to do. The question is: Who do we turn to and where do we go for clarity of information?

I am convinced that we must return to our Father's wisdom. Let me explain. Luke's gospel, chapter 15, reveals the story of a certain man who had two sons. The younger son told his father to give him his part of the family inheritance. This younger son took his part, left home and went to a far country where he squandered his wealth. He left the wisdom of his father and operated with a wisdom that was not conducive to his well-being.

"And he [Jesus] said, A certain man had two sons: And the younger of them said to his father, Father, give me the portion of goods that falleth to me. And he divided them unto them his living. And not many days after the younger son gathered all together, and took his journey into a far country, and there wasted his substance with riot-ous living." Luke 15:11-13

This young man figured he knew enough that he no longer needed the wisdom of his father. He disconnected himself from his father. He made no attempt to contact his father. He was his own man and didn't want anyone telling him what to do. Believe it or not, herein lies the root cause of so many health problems, including being overweight and obese. Let's face it--most Americans are born without an ailment. The majority of physical problems are developed, not inherited.

If you believe the lie that most of our physical problems were inherited, then you'll never get to the root cause of disease. To say that most health problems are inherited takes us out of the "driver's seat" and puts us into the back seat. Meaning we have little or no control over what may happen to us. I'm not denying diseases that have been inherited, but even then there is hope. Hear me clearly, most health problems are not inherited; they are developed.

If health problems develop, it follows that the individual has a part to play in their development, consciously or unconsciously. But there's good news in what I've just said. The good news is that you don't have to remain a victim but can become a victor. In other words, take responsibility for what happens. Take charge. Stop being a passive listener, a passive receiver and a passive eater.

When I go to restaurants, I get aggressive about the menu. I don't just go along with what's put before me without asking questions. It's my life. I'm paying for the food and I have a right to ask questions in the interest of my health. I see too many people eat in a manner I call "passively." Example: If bread is on the menu, I ask if there is wheat bread available to replace the white bread. Or I may ask if sourdough bread is available. I may also ask for extra vegetables instead of the white rice that comes with the dish. Or I may ask that my bread be not toasted and given to me plain. This may sound nit-picky, yet it can make the difference in good health or bad weight problems or the maintaining of an ideal weight.

Back to the prodigal son. The prodigal son disconnected himself from the wisdom of his father. Had he stayed connected, he would have known how to wisely use the part of the inheritance that belonged to him. Well, we've done the same thing in the area of nutrition, wellness and weight control. We've left the wisdom of God--concerning what to put in the body and how to take care of it--and have done our own thing. Therefore, we've reaped the weight problems we have today.

I don't believe the problem is as complicated as it has been advertised to be. Certain advertisements keep us thinking that our weight problems are purely genetic. If we keep thinking that way, then we will continue to ignore our need to change your eating habits and rely on medications or surgical procedures. We are then bent to respond to the solutions of the advertisers. If they can convince you that all weight problems are inherited and that they have a solution to your inherited weight problem, then you buy into their solution and whatever they're selling. They can make money off of your ignorance about the root cause of your weight problem. I'm simply saying, let's *"go back home"* to the wisdom of our creator about what to eat, how to lose weight and how to keep it off.

State of the Weight

Americans are getting fatter and fatter. Consequently weight concerns have become a major focal point among the general public. We are now entertained by exercise shows from the early morning hours throughout the day. Pharmaceutical companies are advertising more drugs that claim to promote weight loss. Walking trails are constantly being developed. And there is a plethora of exercise equipment constantly being developed--all to help combat the overwhelming weight issues plaguing today's fat Americans.

In an article released August 19, 2002, US News and World Report addressed the weight problems among US adults and children.

> *"America has become a fat nation. More than 61 percent of adults are overweight, and 27 percent of them--50 million people--are obese, according to the U.S. Surgeon General's report released last December. In the next decade, weight-related illnesses threaten to overwhelm the health care system. New evidence from the Framingham Heart Study shows that obesity doubles the risk of heart failure in women. A man with 22 extra pounds has a 75 percent greater chance of having a heart attack than one at a healthy weight. Gaining just 11 to 18 pounds doubles the risk of developing Type II diabetes--an illness that has increased by nearly 50 percent in only the past decade.*

Weight is also taking a heavy toll on the nation's children. The percentage of 6-to-11 year-olds who are overweight has nearly doubled in two decades, and for adolescents the percentage has tripled. Pediatricians are treating conditions rarely before diagnosed in young people. In a recent study of 813 overweight Louisiana school children, for example, 58 percent had at least one heart-disease risk factor, such as high-blood pressure, cholesterol, or insulin levels. Four percent of adolescents now have "adult onset" (or Type II) diabetes, and in some clinics teens represent half of all new cases."

According to the above statements, we can no longer sit back and be passive concerning our weight issues. We must be pro-active and get to the root causes that are threatening our well-being, as well as our national wallets. We are spending more on health care than some nations have in their total budget. And much of what we are spending on health care is in response to weight related problems.

Let's look at a few of the contributing factors to the problems of being overweight and obese. First, I believe we are eating too much. Like Sodom (Ezekiel 16:49), we eat too much and exercise too little. We simply put in more than we burn off.

Decades ago, many Americans worked jobs that required a lot of physical labor. Today, much of that physical labor has been replaced with technology. So, for the most part, we don't move as much now as we did then. Yet we are eating more. When you go to many fast food restaurants, you are served super size portions or you have access to all-you-can-eat buffets. The attitude of many seems to be, *"I will eat my money's worth"* without any regard for the end result of such a mentality. We are being wooed with food in shopping malls, in our schools, and at many social events--especially at church.

Secondly, we are eating foods loaded with chemicals and preservatives that constipate our systems, leading to more weight problems. Finally, our children don't exercise today as children have done in the past. Physical exercise is not stressed in schools as it used to be. Nowadays our children come home and are entertained by television and video games rather than being outside, riding bicycles or playing ball games.

A Disastrous Diet

So many people's diets are so drastic that they would almost have to kill themselves to lose weight and keep it off. I talked with a lady a few years ago who said she wanted to lose a hundred pounds before her wedding. The first thing I told her was to fax me a copy of what she eats on a somewhat regular basis (on a given day). What she sent me is what I classified as a disastrous diet. Here is what she sent me.

Morning
2 eggs – fried
Bacon or pan sausage

2 slices of toast
milk or coffee (with sugar & crème)

Lunch
Hamburger, chips, soda or
Ham & cheese (wheat bread),
chips, soda

Dinner
Fried chicken or pork chops
Whole corn or rice & gravy
Potatoes
Greens and/or yams

Late Night
Cereal & milk
Peanut butter sandwich

Notice that she had no fruit in her diet. Fruit operates as a cleansing agent for the body. Eating fruit nurtures the cells and helps keep bowel movements regular. The more regular your bowel movements are, the less your risk of maintaining unwanted pounds. The vegetables she ate were all cooked. There was no water in the information she sent me (although she drank some, from what she told me verbally). She said she just didn't like water. I've heard this all too often, from many people.

Reasons Why People are Overweight

First of all, people are overweight because of eating diets dominated with cooked foods. I am not against cooked foods. I eat them myself. However, cooked foods don't pass through your digestive system as quickly as raw food. Many people over cook their foods, killing all the enzymes and destroying the fiber.

When this occurs, the transit time of the food in the bowels is slower. The longer the food stays in you, the greater the chance for weight gain. Furthermore, the longer you cook the food, the more nutrients you lose. The more nutrients you lose, the more food you will want because you were not physiologically satisfied. Nothing satisfies hunger like raw food. I'm not talking about merely filling space in your intestines; I'm talking about nurturing your cells to the point that they stop crying for more food. When the body is satisfied, it won't keep asking for more. So then, the more nutritious your meals are, the less food your body will require. The less nutritious, the more your body will require. The more it requires, the greater your chance for weight gain.

I once talked with a gentleman who asked me about advice on losing weight. I asked him, "How much raw food do you eat daily (on a scale of 1 to 10: 10 being the highest)?" He told me none! He was about 80 pounds overweight. I told him he could lose the weight if he started to exercise (which he was not doing at the time), but, unless he changed his diet, too, he would have to work harder because it takes more energy to break down cooked foods than raw foods.

Secondly, people are overweight because of overeating. Next time you dine out, glance at the plate of the average person and you'll see that he or she is overeating. Many people eat as if there is no tomorrow. They eat as if it is their last meal. Then there are those who eat too much of a certain kind of food. For example the individual who has two or three kinds of meats on his plate, but only one vegetable On one occasion I talked to a gentleman who told me he rarely ate vegetables (cooked or raw). There was no wonder why he was having weight problems and hemorrhoids.

Overeating causes three major problems. First of all, it confuses our metabolism. The body can only breakdown a certain amount of food at one time. When we overeat, we have food backed up or put "on hold" for digestion. The longer the food has to wait for digestion, the greater the chances for developing gases and creating other ailments. Secondly, overeating makes you overweight. Why? Because the longer the food stays in you, the more likely that it turns into fat. Overeating leads to being overweight, and being overweight leads to a desire to want to eat more. There are numerous reasons for this, both psychological and physiological, ranging from personal insecurities to outright addictions.

Thirdly, overeating increases the likelihood of diseases such as heart disease, certain cancers, diabetes, and hypertension. Keep in mind that every action has a reaction. You can't overeat and think nothing is going to happen in your body. It is better (if you need to) to eat more times in a day (eating smaller quantities of food) than to eat once or twice, eating larger quantities of food. Smaller meals keep the stomach from becoming stretched. Smaller meals also help to raise the metabolism. Both of these are important factors regarding obesity.

The third reason why people are overweight is a lack of discipline. It means you consume food without restraints. The bible calls it being a glutton. A disciplined individual says "after a certain amount of food, I will stop." To consistently eat beyond that certain amount of food is to develop a habit that leads to continual weight gain or at least a struggle to keep the body's weight in check. To be disciplined means we must stop excusing or pitying ourselves. We must hold ourselves responsible to a higher standard than anybody else expects of us. Being disciplined means we don't flow with the tide that everyone else is flowing with. The following scripture depicts the kind of discipline needed to maintain a healthy life and an ideal weight.

"Enter ye in at the strait (disciplined, difficult) gate: for wide is the gate, and broad is the way, which leadeth to destruction (sickness and disease), and many those be which go in thereof: But straight is the gate and narrow is the way, which leadeth unto life, and few there be that find it." Matthew 7:13-14

The fourth reason people are overwehgit is that they are eating dead foods. Today there is so much deception as far as food is concerned. People are eating more food void of life elements than ever before. They are eating foods that have no enzymes, water, fiber and very little, if any, vitamins and minerals. These foods are often man-made foods (foods that have been processed, refined, genetically modified or simply made from man-made chemicals).

Foods that have no life in them strain our digestive system, cause havoc on our nervous system and slow down our circulatory system. With this "lifeless" kind of food, weight struggles are destined to be. It takes life to reproduce life. This is a law that can be clearly understood. Yet people continue to eat stripped, processed, refined dead foods that cannot reproduce life. Let's stop deceiving ourselves, thinking we can get from man-made foods only what God-made foods can produce.

The fifth reason why people are overweight is excessive eating of *"sweets."* Eating excessive desserts contributes to weight gain. Desserts are a part of most people's meals. To some it is a major part of their meal. I personally love desserts and have loved them all my life. A problem arises when we habitually eat two or three desserts in one meal or snack on desserts throughout the day.

Desserts carry what nutritionist call "empty calories." They carry little, if any nutrients. Of course, they are usually sweet and tickle the taste buds. I have often seen some people eat their desserts before eating their main course. Eating desserts first leads directly to weight gain because we fill up on these foods that are usually void of fiber (the colon sweeping element) and loaded with sugar and other substances that cause weight problems. To stop weight gain through the avenue of desserts, we need to simply make wiser choices.

Consider desserts other than pies, cakes, ice cream and candy. I have trained myself to love raisins, dates, tofutti (a non-dairy, no fat and low cholesterol soy product that tastes like ice cream) and other naturally sweet desserts. You'll have to shop around to find what you like. Be creative, try something different, but whatever you do, break the dessert habit that will ruin your health and creates weight gain.

Another reason for over-eating is food advertisements. Food advertisements contribute to weight problems. There's hardly a place you can go nowadays where there's not a lot of food advertisements. You see them on television scores of times a day. When you go to the movies you see them. They are at ball games, in our malls, in drug stores, on billboards and just so many places. Because food is advertised so much, it stays on our minds. As a result we tend to want to eat even when we aren't hungry. Again, this leads to weight problems. We simply have to be aware that food companies are trying to get us to eat more so their sales will increase. Don't be fooled, food companies are not looking out for your health; they are pushing sales to satisfy the stockholders of their companies.

The seventh reason is that we are trying to eat "our money's worth" from buffets. Your stomach and intestines can hold only a certain amount of food. When you go over that amount, your body, instinctively alerts you to what you have done. Like many, I used to have the mentality that I would eat my money's worth when I went to a restaurant that served buffet style foods. Show me an individual who does this three or four times a week, and I'll show you someone who will probably have pounds multiplied instead of merely added on.

Our attitude towards a buffet should be that we have more of a variety to choose from rather than an access to more to consume. Eating super sized meals fits into this category as well. People think *"Wow! I can get more for my money by purchasing the super sized meal."* Let me remind you that fast food restaurants sell you the super size as a tactic to play on your thinking. They know that if you can be convinced that you are getting more for your money, you'll keep coming back. But what is the super sized meal doing to your waistline and your health? The super size meals, like the regular sized meals are usually loaded with chemicals that make you hungrier and fatter, and worst of all, they are usually void of the necessary nutrients that sustain optimum health.

Reason number eight is eating to fill an emotional void, which can lead to unnecessary eating. We are often unconscious to what we do when we get upset, depressed, have a disappointing day or go through some other emotionally challenging moment. Of course everyone responds differently to life's ordeals. Some people eat to comfort themselves. They are no different from the individual who drinks or smokes when faced with disturbing moments. Eating is used as a pacifier to fill an emotional void. Here's why building strong, supporting relationships is so important. In times of crisis, you need to lean more on people than on food, if your tendency is to eat a lot during these times.

The last reason is eating heavy meals at night assures an increase in weight. If you are already dealing with a slow metabolism, then eating late at night (especially heavy meals) compounds the problem. After a certain time in the evening, the body slows down. Eating late at night causes the body to have to work outside of the hours it was designed to work. Think of how you feel when you are expecting to get off at five o'clock, but your boss informs you at 4:30 p.m. that he needs you to work over until 6:00 or 6:30 p.m. – and this happens several days in a row. You exhaust yourself with the extra hours. So it is when we eat late at night. The body is ready to rest, but we tell it to keep digesting. We bring confusion and chaos to its design. The end result is weight gain.

Health & Wellness Nuggets

- Weight loss is made easy when we return to our Maker's wisdom about nutrition.

- Many physical problems are developed, not inherited.

- Good health begins with your acceptance of responsibility for your well-being.

- The reason many people are overweight is that they eat too much and exercise too little.

- You can't eat just anything and expect to keep your weight down.

- God did not put ingredients in our food supply that would make us fat.

- The ingredients in man-made foods make you hungrier and fatter.

- Consistent weight maintenance is the result of a lifestyle, not a diet plan.

- The more regular your bowel movements, the less chance you have of gaining weight.

- People are overweight because of overeating.

Health & Wellness

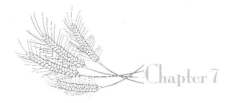

Chapter 7

The Value Of Exercise

"And the Lord God took the man, and put him into the Garden of Eden to dress it and to keep it." (Genesis 2:15)

For years I've listened to many Christians who downplayed the value of exercise by misunderstanding the scriptures. As you look closely at the above scripture, you will see that exercise (or work) was instituted by God for man's physical well-being as well as other reasons. A key scripture that was used for years in Christendom was I Timothy 4:8 which says, *"For bodily exercise profiteth little; but godliness is profitable unto all things."* Many people have aged faster and died prematurely because of not understanding this scripture.

The bible was not saying that there is no benefit in exercise or work. Solomon declared in Proverbs 14:23, *"In all labor (exercise) there is profit."* What Paul was saying in I Timothy 4:8 was that in comparison to spiritual things, physical exercise would be secondary. However, when it comes to physical things or the physical dimension of man and his well-being, physical activity greatly matters.

Except in sporting events, there was not so much emphasis on bodily exercise generations ago. Why? Because the average individual worked manually in fields or factories. Today tractors, trucks, harvesting machines and computers have replaced manual work. People are sitting behind desks now when then people were out in the fields. Thus, there is the need for exercise programs and regimens to help keep the body in good physical condition. Today there are many physical fitness cassettes, videos, and workout groups offered around our country and the world. Physical health requires a balance between diet and nutrition, exercise and proper rest. The Lord established all of these to be a part of a cycle that would promote healthy and vibrant living.

As a lover of sports, I understand how vital it is to have some daily regime of exercise, especially if you are regularly involved in sporting competitions. Even if you are a sports spectator fanatic, health authorities have been telling you for years that you should exercise to have good health. According to the Centers for Disease Control, about 4 out of 5 adults get little or no exercise. There's no mystery why our joints are stiffening, why we so easily pull a muscle, feel fatigued or age faster than the preceding generation. We simply are not giving our bodies enough exercise, if any at all.

Many people are coming home from an office job or a job where there is not a lot of physical labor involved, flopping down in front of a television for hours and slowly inviting poor health due to a lack of physical exercise--plus poor eating habits. Many people don't know that exercise is one of the biblical foundations to good health. Exercise will help prevent disease and sustain vibrant living. Let's examine some of the healing, physical, and emotional benefits of exercise.

Studies have shown that people who exercise pay half the medical bills and have one-third the number of sick days as people who
don't. I observed this firsthand when working at a state prison for
twelve years. That job had no physical labor involved. Sadly, the
majority of correctional officers I worked with were not just overweight, but grossly overweight. Usually all we had to do all day
long was to watch and supervise the inmates. If you did not have
some physical regime of your own, then you were doomed to catch
a disease known among correctional officers as the "done-lopped
disease". This meant that your stomach had grown so big (because
of being overweight) that it had "done lopped" over your belt.

Through my visits to the hospital and having known family members and friends who have had various illnesses, I have noticed that
doctors often put patients on a physical regime to help speed up the
healing process.   A study at the University of North Carolina at
Chapel Hill showed that an inactive person's risk of heart disease is
the same as that of someone who smokes a pack of cigarettes a day.
As far as healing is concerned, exercise also--

reduces fat
Those who exercise become leaner. Cancer thrives more   readily
in fatty tissue than lean tissue.

reduces constipation
Constipation has been linked with colon cancer and inactive people
are more likely to be constipated. Exercise stimulates the peristaltic
action of the intestines, which results in regular and more frequent
bowel movements.

increases blood flow
Small arteries can begin to shut down through lack of physical activity. Exercise expands and re-opens these blood vessels. It is the
flow of blood that oxygenates your body and carries away wastes.

So exercise both detoxifies your system and oxygenates your cells. Exercise also burns away excess weight, lowers blood pressure, improves the cholesterol profile, improves blood sugar and insulin dynamics, helps prevent bone-thinning osteoporosis, helps alleviate chronic lower back pain, and improves immune function, moods and mental performance.

Another benefit of exercise is the physical value. Since my grammar and high school days on the track and football teams, I have always maintained a desire to stay *"physically fit."* To this day if my wife says, *"Honey, it looks like your stomach is getting round,"* I go into a frenzy. I refuse to sit back and allow excessive pounds to embrace me or to picture myself drying up into old age slowly. Furthermore, I don't believe we have to look like a prune the older we get.

I have observed the life of people like Dr. Norman W. Walker, who gave us the testimony of a vibrant life for over a hundred years. From a physical value, exercise promotes one of man's basic needs for life--oxygen. Oxygen is the "breath of life" that God breathed into Adam at the creation. Our bodies are made up of trillions of cells. Each cell has its own entity and is capable of reproducing itself. However, in order to sustain life and reproduce itself, a cell has specific needs that must be met. These basic needs are an adequate food supply and an effective waste disposal system.

The quality of our food supply along with the efficiency of the waste disposal system will determine the quality and length of our lives. Most sicknesses, in whatever form they manifest themselves (whether colds, flu, diabetes, heart attacks, etc.) are the result of our failing to provide our cells with the proper building materials and or failing to adequately remove the toxic wastes from the cells.

One of the greatest needs the body has is for pure air. Shortness of breath is something many Americans suffer with. Why? Because we are not getting enough exercise, if any. In his book, God's Way to Ultimate Health, Dr. George Malkmus gives some potent facts about oxygen:

1. The quality of the air (its purity) we breathe affects the quality and length of the life we live. Breathing good clean air increases the quality and length of our life. Breathing polluted air decreases the quality and length of life!

2. Increase the supply of oxygen to the brain (through deep breathing and exercise) and mental abilities will increase and the brain will become more alert! Decrease the supply of oxygen to the brain (through smoking, air pollution, and a sedentary life) and the brain's mental abilities will decrease and become sluggish. Cut off oxygen supply to the brain for only a brief moment (as during a stroke) and parts of the brain will die, producing paralysis in various parts of the body.

3. Increase the supply of oxygen to the body's cells and the body becomes full of energy and life! Decrease the supply of oxygen to the cells and the body fails to provide the energy necessary to perform properly. Then we begin to feel tired, sluggish, and listless.

4. An increase in the supply of oxygen to the body's cells helps us mentally and emotionally and we become happy and optimistic. Decrease the supply of oxygen to the body's cells and we become discouraged, depressed, and pessimistic.

5. Increase the supply of oxygen to the body's cells and sickness cannot find a foothold. Decrease the supply of oxygen and the body's cells provide the breeding ground for sickness. Sickness and disease cannot survive in an aerobic (oxygenated) atmosphere.

There's no doubt about it, if the body is going to stay healthy, then we must get sufficient oxygen for its proper functioning. We must, therefore, have regular times of exercising with an understanding of its physical benefits.

Lastly, there are the emotional benefits that come from exercise. Let me say that the emotions play an extremely important part in the psychological and physical well being of an individual. We have heard the statement for years that your "attitude determines your altitude" (or how successful you become in life). Our society has been plagued with emotional problems from deep depression to suicide. We must understand that if the body isn't getting the exercise it needs, emotional problems can arise.

When you exercise, chemicals call endorphins (anti-depressants) are released into your body and you, therefore, begin to experience a sense of well-being. Notice that when you go for long periods of time without exercise, not only do you not feel physically pepped, you also lose that emotional well-being. I have personally taken note of the emotional high that comes from my aerobic exercise. Since I have learned about endorphins and experienced firsthand the sensations I get from aerobic exercise, I now love to do what I used to despise.

I used to enjoy the exercise that I got only when in competitive sports. The reason I'm mentioning this is because I know that there are some of you who could care not less about a lot of exercising. But the advantages are overwhelming. First of all, it does not take a whole lot. A little bit (consistently done) will significantly promote well being. Secondly, when you begin to renew your mind to the emotional and physical benefits exercise gives to you, this will help you have a greater sense of appreciation for exercise.

Exercise then works as an anti-depressant, enabling you to handle stress more effectively. As quoted from Walking for Health by Mark Bricklin and Maggie Spilner:

"Both fit and unfit people were subjected to the mental stress of an arithmetic test. Meanwhile, researchers at the University of Toronto monitored both the rate and the electrical activity of their hearts."

"Even with this mild challenge, we saw a reliable difference in the electrical activity of the heart," wrote John Fuody, PH.D, head of the laboratory where the study was run. He goes on to say, *"The change was in the amplitude of the heart's T wave. This wave occurs when the heart is pumping and pulling new blood in. The change indicated that in less fit people, the heart overreacted to "fight" or "flight" biochemicals--such as adrenalin--that are produced during psychological stress."*

By using our bodies the way they were meant to be used, we can free ourselves from stress and fatigue while boosting our immune systems and conditioning our hearts and lungs. It will do us well if we simply plan a physical regime and be determined to be consistent with it. Please be advised that a variety of exercises will be needed to ensure the building of your strength, flexibility, and overall balanced fitness. In other words, just doing push-ups or sit-ups alone won't give you the workout needed to sustain vibrant health. You must develop an exercise routine that really suits you.

Don't try to fit into someone else's mode. Exercising must be fun to you or else you will not continue to do something that you don't enjoy. Remember that every system in you body – circulatory, digestive, respiratory, nervous, skeletal, and muscular--works at top effectiveness when you have regular exercise. Regular exercise will help prevent many diseases. Don't become complacent because of our modern conveniences. If we are going to survive and live long lives, then we must keep our bodies active. Your body was designed for activity.

In his book The Most Dangerous Sport, Dr. G.A. Sheehan, M.D. stated, "We are constantly being warned to check with our physicians before beginning athletics. What we are not told are the risks of not being athletic--that the most dangerous sport of all is watching it from the stands. The weakest among us can become some kind of athlete, but only the strongest survive as spectators. Only the hardiest can withstand the perils of inertia, inactivity, and immobility. Man was not made to remain at rest."

Health & Wellness Nuggets

- Exercise aids in bowel movement.

- Exercise increases blood flow.

- Exercise lowers blood pressure.

- Exercise enhances the immune system.

- Exercise improves mood and mental performance

- Exercise works as an anti-depressant, enabling you to handle stress more effectively.

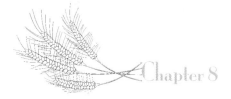

Chapter 8

Understanding The Systems Of The Body

"If anything is sacred the human body is sacred."
Walt Whitman

*"Whose property is my body? Probably mine. I so regard it.
If I experiment with it, who must be answerable? I, not the State.
If I choose unjudiciously, does the State die? Oh, no."*
Mark Twain

If you believe what the above authors have stated, it is imperative that we study, understand and contribute wisely to the development and protection of our bodies. Our health is our number one wealth. If we are not feeling well, then nothing matters more to us than getting better. Most of our physical problems can be stopped before developing if we understand the body's organs and systems and their role in our physical well-being. Notice that I also said that disease is something that is developed. Few people relative to the whole population are born with a disease. Furthermore, sickness and disease don't suddenly strike you like a rattlesnake. Sickness and disease develop, depending on how we habitually deal with our bodies.

Knowledge creates awareness, and awareness develops sensitivity. In this chapter, I will be sharing with you some information about organs and systems of the body. This information is by no means exhaustive. My prayer is that as you study this chapter (as well as the book), your passion to know your body and how best to take care of it will increase to the point that you will study even more. Remember what the scriptures have taught us: *"For where your treasure is, there will your heart be also"* (Matthew 6:21).

We must focus our heart on the treasure of our bodies. We have only one body, and how well it functions is dependent on us. Your body is your responsibility, not your doctor's. If we are going to be responsible for the body God gave us, then we need to study it, know what it takes to effectively function and work with it instead of against it.

Eliminative System

This system is responsible for the removal of toxins and waste out of the body. The major channels of elimination are the colon, skin, urinary and lymph systems. When one or more of these channels aren't functioning well, the others are forced to overwork. If the other channels are unable to handle the overload, then toxins are re-circulated back into the bloodstream and dumped into the weakest organs and tissues of the body. It's like having the commode in your bathroom to overflow. We all know how messy, ugly and smelly this can be. A lack of variety in our diet can cause digestive problems that result in the development of more toxins. Without sufficient elimination of waste, the blood cannot remain clean, thereby causing toxic materials to be re-circulated in the body.

1. Colon

The colon is the sewage system of the body. It is the place where all foods are broken down for distribution of their nutrients to the various parts of the body. It is the breeding ground for bacteria, since it is the place where so much work is done in decomposing food and distributing nutrients, as well as ridding the body of waste.

2. Lungs

The lungs are located in the chest area in the thoracic cavity. Their primary responsibility is the exchanging of gas using the blood and lymph. It is wise to exercise regularly, at least three to five times weekly, giving the body deep breathing in order to pull in the fresh oxygen needed for the lungs to do their job. Keep in mind that the lungs need fresh air – from the outdoors. Today much of the air that many get is re-circulated air from the buildings they work in, the cars they drive and the closed-in homes they live in. Unlike our ancestors, many of us sleep with our windows down through every season of the year.

3. Bronchial Tubes

These are the major air passages in the lungs. The gas exchange takes place at the end of the bronchial tubes.

4. Kidneys

The kidneys are located in the diaphragm region of our anatomy. They are about four inches long, about two inches wide and about one inch thick. They are responsible for regulating the water content of the body, removing wastes and acids from the body, producing and removing urine from the body. Because of the nature of excretions which pass through the kidneys, they are particularly susceptible to infections. Without great amounts of water going through the kidneys, they can't do the job they were designed to do. After considering the amounts of tea, coffee and sodas many people drink, we can truly say it's by the grace of God they have lived as long s they have. Drinking two to three glasses of cranberry tea (preferably without sugar) does wonders for your kidneys.

5. Skin

The skin is the largest organ in the body. It is called by some the "third kidney" because it removes acids from the blood. It excretes water and salt. It protects the body from bacteria invasion and relieves the kidneys by sweating, which removes toxins, mineral wastes and acids. Through our skin, we put all sorts of toxins that we don't recognize are damaging. For years I've rubbed deodorant sticks under my arms, failing to realize those sticks contained aluminum and other unnatural substances in them. Aluminum is a contributing substance to Alzheimer's disease.

A good rule to go by is "If you can't put it in your mouth, then don't put it on your skin." If we would eat more foods containing silicon, iron, potassium, vitamins A, B and niacin, we wouldn't need so many cosmetics to cover up skin defects. Such foods are apples, bananas, beans, corn, cucumbers, spinach, and onions, to name a few. Due to a lack of nutrients, years ago, I had acne spots in various places on my body. When I changed my diet to include more fruits and vegetables, the spots went away. The key to healthy skin is a nutritious diet.

6. Lymph Glands

The lymph glands make up the largest content of fluid in the body and carry more waste than the blood. Every cell and tissue in the body is constantly bathed in the lymph fluid. Lymph fluid penetrates areas too small for blood vessels and operates in the conversion of food to lymph fluid which enters the blood stream.

These glands are a major part of the body's transportation system. Without the proper amount of water needed for the body, these glands couldn't do their job. Also without essential nutrients such as iodine, potassium, calcium and magnesium, the lymph glands are limited in their functioning capacity. Lymph nodes are at certain places in the lymphatic system. The lymph nodes supply lymphocytes (white blood cells formed in the lymphoid tissue) to the circulatory system and work to remove bacteria and foreign particles from the lymph. Nodes are in the armpits, groin, neck, inner thighs or in the fatty part of the bowel. A few years ago before I started using natural deodorant, I used to have swellings under my armpits (in the lymph nodes) from the deodorant I was using. When I changed from the deodorants containing aluminum and other man-made chemicals, the swelling left and hasn't come back since. Be careful about what you put on your skin because it eventually gets into your lymph system and blood stream.

The Breathing and Respiratory System

Some of the organs that comprise the respiratory system are the lungs (which we discussed in the eliminative system) bronchi, pleura and trachea. On this system, we will be looking at the system as a whole, more so than the individual organs. This system functions to bring oxygen to and remove carbon dioxide from the blood. The atmosphere of any city is loaded with carbon monoxide (the deadly exhaust from engines), gasoline, kerosenes and other similar products that are responsible for many respiratory ailments and pollution of the blood.

The value of fresh air (oxygen) can not be underestimated in its role in the breathing and respiratory system. Oxygen is the first nutrient in the body and you can live only a few minutes wihout it. Oxygen

enhances life by strengthening metabolism and regenerative functions. It also kills bacteria. Simply put, the optimal functioning of
our breathing and respiratory system is dependent on the oxygen
flowing through our bodies.

The Glandular System

1. Adrenals

The adrenals are located on the top of the kidneys. They are responsible for the metabolism of carbohydrates and the regulation of
blood sugar. They maintain the body's equilibrium and speed up the
body's metabolism when it's under stress. These glands are probably more frequently exhausted in the stress of life than any other
gland. The exhaustion of these glands brings low blood pressure,
loss of energy and lack of the will to face and overcome stress. The
adrenal glands benefit from rest and relaxation. Without proper rest,
the body doesn't have the chance to recharge itself with energy for
the next day's activities. Rest enables the body to repair and rebuild
its cells.

2. Pituitary

The pituitary is responsible for growth hormone production, thyroid
and adrenal stimulation and regulation. It is also responsible for
ovary and testes regulation, sex drive and reproductive activities.
Keep in mind that without proper nutrition and exercise, none of
these organs can do the job it was designed to do.

3. Thyroid

The thyroid is located at the front and sides of the neck. Some of its
responsibilities are to increase blood sugar and blood sugar regulation, lower blood calcium by depositing the calcium in the bones
and to stimulate the cells to break down protein for energy. Iodine is

the most important nutrient in the proper functioning of the thyroid gland. A goiter (enlargement) of the thyroid, visible at the front of the neck, results from a deficiency of iodine.

Some years ago I observed that the thyroid gland on the right side of my wife's neck was swelling. I went to a health food store, bought some kelp (which contains iodine) and gave her a half of teaspoon of it. Within two days, the swelling had gone completely down. She was lacking iodine in her diet. Had the swelling continued, she would have had a big goiter on her neck. A diet lacking iodine weakens the thyroid function. Refined and processed foods remove iodine as well as other nutrients. The lack of iodine contributes to retarded growth in children, bad teeth, dull mental faculties, weak metabolism and poor elimination. Foods rich in iodine are blueberries, carrots, cucumbers, fish, garlic, kale, and tomatoes, to name a few.

4. Pancreas

The pancreas is a very important gland in our body that should be given great respect. It regulates the blood sugar level by releasing the hormone insulin from a part of the pancreas known as the islands of Langerhans. When the body is toxic and the colon is troubled with fermented and putrefied waste, then these glands are unable to produce the insulin. This results in an intolerance of sugar by the body. Thus the volume of sugar is increased and released into the kidneys. This results in a condition we know all too well as sugar diabetes.

A chronic pancreatic problem which leads to diabetes is unlike most diseases associated with diet. A diet high in foods that have been processed, refined and low in fiber is believed to be behind certain types of diabetes. Pancreatic juice contains digestive enzymes which help to establish the right conditions for the intestinal enzymes to do their job in the small intestine.

5. Other Glands

Other glands in this system include the thymus gland, responsible for growth and sexual development and the stimulation of antibody production; the ovaries, responsible for ovulation and the production of hormones; the testes, responsible for sperm production, secretion of testosterone and regulation of sexual behavior; and the pineal gland, which plays an active role in health and wellness on the mental and physical plane. It is sensitive to light and is stimulated by the sun's rays. Known as the "peace" gland, it influences our sleep-wake pattern and plays a major role in rest, relaxation and healing. Open your blinds and let the Sun come in.

The Reproductive System

Of course we can readily understand that this system is responsible for the body's ability to reproduce. The organs in this system are the uterus, vagina, mammary glands, prostate, ovaries and testes, and the penis. From a nutritional standpoint, what feeds the sexual glands also feeds the nerves and brain. Foods high in lecithin promote better nerve function and better sexual gland functioning. Even the protective sheaths around the brain are composed of lecithin. Lecithin improves brain functioning, protects against heart disease and aids in the absorption of thiamin and vitamin A.

The Digestive System

The digestive system is basically a long tube beginning at the mouth and ending at the anus. Its purpose is to break down food (mechanically and chemically), so it can eventually be carried by the blood and lymph into the cells for usage. The body can only build, repair and sustain itself with the food and drink we give it.

Your body was designed to thrive off a wide range of items provided by God for it. Note that I said provided by God and not by man. Eating a devitalized diet leads to a devitalized life and poor health. God did not design the body to live off of chemical additives, preservatives, flavorings, artificial colorings and so forth that many of our foods today are loaded with. We must ask ourselves the question, "Will this food promote or hurt my health?"

Remember, for every action, there is a reaction. You reap what you sow; you are what you eat. To value the human life is to gain knowledge and understanding of what's right for good health. I've come to realize that it's not just what you eat, but what you are able to digest and assimilate. The digestive system provides nutrients the body needs to function. Depending on what you give your body, it will produce vibrant health and long life or struggles with ailments, sickness and disease and a premature death. Let's get real, you can't eat junk food and expect your body to produce a miracle. Stop! Think about what you are putting into your mouth and how you are treating your body overall.

1. The Stomach: The stomach is like a laboratory. It is the first major organ in the digestive system. It releases gastric enzymes and hydrochloric acid for the break down of foods. It churns and breaks the food down to mix it with the gastric juices. Also the stomach regulates the flow of food into the intestines.

2. Pancreas: It regulates the blood sugar level by releasing the hormone insulin.

3.   Liver: The liver is the largest gland in the body and is the organ that carries on the most active and extensive operation in the anatomy. The liver detoxifies the body's acids and metabolic wastes. Its most important function is secreting bile which is used to digest fats. The typical American diet is damaging the liver. Why? Because of such poor choices as refined white flour products, processed and imitation foods, and refined foods that have been stripped of natural vitamins, minerals and enzymes. Cumulative toxins (such as insecticides and preservatives) also affect the liver's ability to function properly.

Probably the most common cause of liver malfunction is overeating. To overeat causes liver fatigue because of the excess work placed on the liver. When it is overworked, it may not detoxify harmful substances properly. Again, diet plays a major role in the well-being and functioning of the liver. Eating a diet consisting of seventy-five percent raw foods greatly limits the chance of liver malfunctioning. Two vegetables that promote liver functioning are beets and carrots. Drinking the juice of these vegetables helps to speed up the process of nurturing the liver.

4.   Gall Bladder: Attached to the underside of the liver is the gall bladder. It serves as storage for the bile secreted from the liver. Bile is important in digestion, especially the digestion of fats. Drinking three tablespoons of olive oil with the juice of a lemon before bed and upon awakening helps to remove gallstones and protect the gallbladder.

5.   Small Intestines: The organ that completes the digestive process is the small intestine. The small intestine produces enzymes for the digestion of carbohydrates, fats and proteins. It breaks down by its peristaltic movement. Again, proper nutrition and exercise assist this organ in fulfilling its role.

The Nervous System

The nervous system is made up of the brain, spinal cord and the nerves. It is an electrical system that connects the brain to the organs. Please note, food in its pure state (raw and void of artificial colors, flavor and preservatives) have electrical impulses that nurture an electrically designed entity called our bodies. The nervous system is the center for consciousness, memory, reasoning and emotions. It monitors our internal and external environment, adjusting the body to maintain a state of balance.

The nervous system is the main communication network of the body. It is one of our most valuable assets. During sleep, the nerve system works like a storage battery to replenish the vital forces and build up the storage of energy. Nerves are the first to sound an alarm when there is anything wrong in the system. Whatever affects the nerves affects the rest of the body. Like the other systems, the nervous system operates off of the food you eat and the liquid you drink. You can't eat refined sugar, fried foods and processed foods and think that your nervous system will operate at maximum capacity. Neither can you drink carbonated, caffeine sodas and get the best performance from the nervous system or any other system or organ of the body. Nutrients that build the nervous system are the B vitamins, vitamin D and E, phosphorus, silicon and calcium.

Not only does what you eat and drink affect the nervous system, but so does rest and sunlight. Notice how we tend to get sleepy after we've been in the sun for a period of time. It's because the sun has a calming, relaxing effect upon our nervous system. Don't be fooled--sunlight is good for you. Sunlight stimulates the nutritive processes of the body in many chronic disorders such as anemia and tuberculosis. Sunlight has also been known to lower blood pressure and cholesterol, kill bacteria and enhance the immune system.

The Circulatory System

The circulatory system consists of the heart, arteries, veins and capillaries which are fluid transportation structures. This system is responsible for transporting blood that carries nutrients to various parts of the body. It also carries away waste from cell metabolism. It is also responsible for the fluid balance in the body.

Blood is the vital liquid transported through the circulatory system. The average human body contains approximately five quarts of blood. There are billions of cells in your blood that travel so fast through your body that you would get dizzy thinking of how fast they move. Their continuous, unobstructed movement is important to your youthfulness and total well-being. Any interference with the blood's health and activity affects your entire body.

The bible declares, *"For the life of the flesh is in the blood"* (Leviticus 17:11). You can say then, "I am only as healthy as my blood." What a statement! However, we must also realize that your blood is only as healthy as the God-prescribed foods you feed it. God did not prescribe anything that would contaminate our blood and cause us to die prematurely. Our problem has been ingesting food items that have been tampered with by man.

Only by eating and drinking natural, live, organic food can the cells be completely nourished--nothing less. We must learn not to be swayed by the opinions and habits of those who have not taken the time to grasp the knowledge of proper nutrition. After all, you stay healthy or start the process of sickness one bite at a time.

Fruits, vegetables, beans and nuts will keep the blood clean and flowing freely through the body, whereas meats, dairy products, preservatives and various types of man-made chemicals defile the blood and prohibit its flow through the body.

Understanding Body Cycles

A few years ago I used to complain a lot about stomach gas and back cramps. I became desperate to find out what was the cause of such pains. Various friends also observed me doing a lot of burping. Well, when I learned what I was doing wrong, I was awestruck. Why? Because this knowledge ran counter to two things I loved to do. Number one was eating plenty of dairy products, and number two was eating anytime I wanted.

We must understand that laws govern life. There are laws that govern our spiritual, mental, physical, social, and financial realms. I was breaking the Law of Body Cycles. I was simply not working with my body in its attempt to handle what I was putting into it!

Hosea the prophet was so correct when he said that God's people are destroyed because of the lack of knowledge. Nutritionalists declare that your body works in cycles to complete the process of handling what you put into it. Your body's cycle works in the following phases: appropriation, assimilation, and elimination.

The appropriation phase is the time when the body is most capable of taking in the foods you serve it. This time frame is usually between 12 p.m. and 8 p.m. The assimilation phase is between 8 p.m. and 4 a.m. This is the time in which your body works to break down and distribute to its various compartments what you have given it.

There was a time I had an unhealthy habit that torments me to this day. I used to love to eat my ice cream and cookies with some sort of chips between 9 p.m. and 12 a.m. and even later. The habit came from my loving to do a lot of reading and research during these wee hours.

The third phase of the body's cycle is the elimination phase. This is the time when the body is saying, "I am most ready to get rid of the wastes and food debris that are not needed." This time frame is from 4 a.m. until noon. Now I know most of you are thinking about breakfast. However, remember the body is most ready to eliminate during this time frame. That doesn't mean that there is no other time during the course of a day where elimination will occur. There are other times and you have experienced them, mainly because of your diet and eating habits coupled with stresses and crisis times.

If you are going to eat breakfast, beware of heavy meals. It is better to eat fresh fruit (which should be governed by your needs so you won't under or over eat) or have some fresh juice. Well, what I did was work on working with my body's cycles. I have since seen the cramps disappear as well as awakened in the morning refreshed instead of feeling as though I had been out in a field working all night long. Your body will tend to register a tired feeling when you eat late at night. Actually, when you work late at night, you offset the process that was designed to keep you psychologically and physically healthy.

Understanding your body cycles will also help you win the war over the battle of the bulge.

Health & Wellness Nuggets

- Disease doesn't strike someone, like a rattlesnake; it is developed.

- Knowledge brings awareness, and awareness develops sensitivity.

- Your body is your responsibility, not your doctor's.

- Rest enables the body to repair and rebuild its cells.

- The digestive system is a long tube beginning at the mouth and ending at the anus.

- Digestion doesn't start in the stomach; it starts in the mouth.

- *"The life of the flesh is in the blood."* (Leviticus 17:11)

Health & Wellness

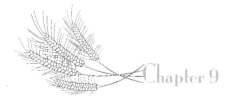

Chapter 9

Herbs And Their Usage

In this chapter, we will discuss how herbs can be used to target the different systems in the body. These systems include the cardiovascular system, the endocrine, nervous and urinary tract system, the digestive and respiratory system, and the structural tissues.

Cardiovascular System

The cardiovascular system includes the blood vessels, circulation, the heart and the lymph nodes. Under each of the following headings are the herbs that can be used to improve the organ, structure and function within the cardiovascular system.

Blood vessels (arteries and veins)	_Heart_
Butcher's broom	Bilberry
Cayenne	Cayenne
Green tea	Garlic
Soy lecithin	Ginkgo
Hawthorn	

Lymph Nodes

Lymph nodes are located throughout the body, but are especially concentrated in the groin and under the arm areas.

Burdock
Dandelion
Garlic
Red clover

Circulation

Cayenne
Garlic
Ginkgo

Endocrine System, Nervous System and Urinary Tract

Endocrine System:

Thymus
Echinacea
Licorice
Stinging nettle

Adrenal Glands
Ginger
Licorice
Rose hips

Pancreas
Cayenne
Green tea
Soy lecithin
Stinging nettle

Nervous System:

Central Nervous System
Chamomile
Ginkgo
Siberian ginseng
Skullcap
Valerian

Brain
Ginger
Ginkgo
Gotu kola
Soy lecithin

Urinary Tract:
Bladder
Butcher's broom
Cranberry
Parsley
Uva ursi

Digestive System and Respiratory System

Digestive Organs:

Liver
Dandelion
Fenugreek
Milk thistle
Garlic
Slippery elm

Intestines
Aloe
Chamomile
Fenugreek

Stomach
Aloe
Chamomile
Garlic
Ginger

Gall Bladder
Barberry
Dandelion

Respiratory Tract:

Lungs
Dong quai
Elderberry
Eucalyptus
Garlic
Ginger
Licorice

Structural Tissues

Hair
Alfalfa
Gingko
Stinging nettle
Sage

Bone
Alfalfa
Rose hips

Skin
Alfalfa
Calendula
Chamomile
Dandelion
Green tea

Joints
Alfalfa
Garlic

Muscle
Horsetail
Stinging nettle

Ears, Eyes and Mouth

Ears
Calendula
Garlic
Gingko
Hyssop

Eyes
Bilberry
Eyebright
Shepherd's purse

Mouth
Goldenseal
Myrrh
Tea tree

HERB USES

HERB	USES
Aloe Vera	*Applied externally*: heals burns, stimulates cell regeneration *Applied internally*: soothes stomach irritation, good for skin and digestive disorders
Barberry	Slows breathing, stimulates intestinal movement
Bilberry	Useful for hypoglycemia, inflammation, stress, anxiety
Black Cohosh	Lowers blood pressure, relieves hot flashes
Black Walnut	Aids digestion, cleanses the body of some types of parasites
Blessed Thistle	Heals the liver, improves circulation, purifies the blood and strengthens the heart
Boneset	Loosens phlegm, reduces fever, calms the body
Buchu	Decreases inflammation of the colon, gums, mucous membrane, prostrate, sinuses
Butcher's Broom	Relieves inflammation, circulatory disorders, varicose veins and vertigo
Calendula	Skin soother, helps to regulate the menstrual cycle and useful for many skin disorders
Cascara Sagrada	Acts as a colon cleanser and as a laxative
Catnip	Aids digestion and sleep, relieves stress, colds and flu
Celery	Reduces blood pressure, good for arthritis and kidney problems
Chamomile	An anti-inflammatory; digestive aid and sleep aid

HERB USES

Cinnamon Counteracts congestion; aids the circulation of the blood; useful disorder problems, diabetes and weight loss

Cranberry Helpful for infections of the urinary tract

Dandelion Improves functioning of the kidneys, pancreas, spleen and stomach; useful for abscesses

Dong Quai Used in treatment of hot flashes, menopausal symptoms and vaginal dryness

Echinacea Good for the immune system; colds and flu

Eucalyptus Clears congestion, has a mild antiseptic action; good for colds and coughs

Eyebright Good for allergies, watery eyes and runny nose

Fennel Promotes the functioning of the kidneys, liver; relieves abdominal pain and gas

Fenugreek Lubricates the intestines; helps asthma and sinus problems by reducing mucus

Garlic Enhances the immune system, lowers blood pressure, improves circulation; Aids in treatment of cancer, colds and flu

Ginger Cleanses the colon, stimulates circulation; useful for bowel disorders, circulatory problems
Note: Can cause stomach distress if taken in large quantities.

Ginkgo Improves brain functioning; headaches, memory loss

Ginseng Diabetes, infertility, lack of energy

Goldenseal Acts as an antibiotic, cleanses the body; improves digestion, and reduces blood pressure

HERB USES

Green Tea	Combats mental fatigue; may lower risk of skin cancer; fights cholesterol buildup
Hops	Good for hyperactivity, pain, toothaches
Horsetail	Useful for gallbladder disorders, inflammation
Hyssop	Relieves congestion, regulates blood pressure, and dispels gas
Irish Moss	Good for many intestinal disorders
Kava Lava	Helpful for anxiety, depression and insomnia
Lavender	Relieves stress and depression; good for headaches
Licorice	Promotes adrenal gland function; beneficial for asthma, chronic fatigue, depression
Milk Thistle	Good for adrenal disorders, inflammatory bowel disorders, weakened immune system
Myrrh	Helps fight harmful bacteria in the mouth; periodontal disease
Papaya	Aids digestion; good for heartburn, indigestion
Parsley	Relieves gas, stimulates normal activity of the digestive system, and freshens breath; helps kidney, bladder, lung, stomach and thyroid function; good for fluid retention, gas, halitosis, high blood pressure, kidney disease, obesity and prostate disorders
Peppermint	Useful for chills, heart trouble, rheumatism
Primrose	Helpful for hot flashes, menstrual problems
Rosemary	Good for headaches and circulatory problems

HERB USES

Sage	Good for hot flashes
St. Johnswort	Good for depression and nerve pain
Saw Palmetto	Good for prostate disorders
Skullcap	Good for anxiety, fatigue, headache, hyperactivity, nervous disorders
Tea Tree	Good for all skin conditions
Thyme	Eliminates gas; lowers cholesterol
Yellow Dock	Acts as a blood purifier and cleanser; good for liver disease and skin disorders

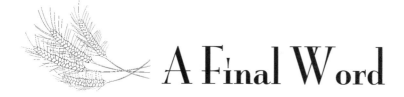

A Final Word

Your health is something you cannot afford to take lightly. If you are going to live healthy, then you must *"take responsibility for your well being."* When you know that patients are out-living their doctors, then definitely we can't afford to let them make decisions about our bodies without our say so. We must educate our children and ourselves. When does all of this education start? I will tell you. It starts with the bible. God is the one who created our magnificent bodies, and in his book is the wisdom that will sustain long life and good health. The psalmist David stated in the book of Psalms chapter 139:14 - 16:

"I will praise thee; for I am fearfully [craftily and carefully] *and wonderfully made: marvelous are thy works and that my soul knoweth right well. My substance was not hid from thee, when I was made in secret, and curiously wrought in the lowest parts of the earth. Thine eyes did see my substance, yet being unperfect and in thy book all my members were written, which in continuance were fashioned, when as yet there was none of them."*

We must simply turn back to God who made us. If we seek his wisdom for our bodies, he will answer us with solutions that will not only heal us, but also keep us well.

Health & Wellness

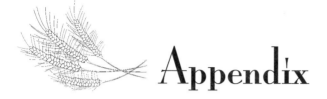

Appendix

Foods to Avoid

1. Soft drinks & diet soda. Replace with organic drinks.
2. Refined sugars. Use all natural, unrefined sugar; honey or Stevia.
3. White bread. Replace with whole wheat bread.
4. Table salt. Replace with Sea Salt.
5. Tea. Replace with caffeine-free herbal teas.
6. White flour products such as: cakes, pies, donuts, etc. Replace with organic, unbleached wheat flour products.
7. Hydrogenated oils or trans fats
8. Processed foods
9. Man-made foods
10. Genetically Modified foods
11. Chlorinated (tap) water
12. Foods with coloring added
13. Foods with Preservatives
14. Homogenized dairy products

Other Things to Avoid

1. Lack of exercise
2. Lack of rest
3. Deodorants. Replace with an organic brand.
4. Lack of sunshine
5. Lack of fresh air
6. Toothpaste with fluoride. Replace with an organic, all-natural brand.
7. Commercial lotions. Replace with an all-natural brand.
8. Perfumes and colognes. Replace with oils, which carry great smells. (As a rule, anything you can't put into your mouth, don't put on your skin.)
9. Holding grudges
10. Revenge
11. Walking out of love with people
12. Speaking negative words
13. Thinking on negative things
14. Stressful music
15. Watching horror movies, especially before sleeping.

Wisdom for Vibrant Health

1. Vibrant, lasting health is developed day by day, meal by meal, and bite by bite.
2. Your number one wealth is your health. Daily invest in it.
3. We must promote health and not merely fight disease.
4. You aren't just what you eat, you are what you assimilate.
5. The body will protest abuse by the indications of pain.
6. Everything that happens in the body is caused by something.
7. Age is no excuse for disease, aches and pains.
8. If it is man-made, don't eat it.

9. Real food will spoil.
10. Read labels.
11. Dominate your food intake with raw foods.

Steps to Greater Health

1. Set a goal for greater health and wellness.
2. Start making changes in your diet, where necessary.
3. Begin an exercise regime if you don't have one. Be consistent with your exercise.
4. Get plenty of sunshine.
5. Eat smaller portions of food.
6. Drink 8 to 10 glasses of water daily.
7. Do a colon cleanse two to three times yearly.
8. Start and develop new relationships.
9. Get a yearly physical.
10. Take yearly vacations.

Healing Scriptures

Psalm 91:16
"With long life will I satisfy him, and shew him my salvation."

Psalm 46:1
"God is our refuge and strength, a very present help in trouble."

Psalm 42:5
"Why art thou cast down, O my soul? and why art thou disquieted in me? hope thou in God: for I shall yet praise Him for the help of his countenance."

Proverbs 3:21-22
"My son, let not them depart from thine eyes: keep sound wisdom and discretion: So shall they be life unto thy soul, and grace to thy neck."

Proverbs 4:20-22
"My son, attend to my words; incline thine ear unto my sayings. Let them not depart from thine eyes; keep them in the midst of thine heart. For they are life unto those that find them, and health to all their flesh."

Proverbs 14:30
"A sound heart is the life of the flesh: but envy the rottenness of the bones."

Psalm 91:1
"He that dwelleth in the secret place of the most High shall abide under the shadow of the Almighty."

II Corinthians 4:18
"While we look not at the things which are seen, but at the things which are not seen: for the things which are seen are temporal; but the things which are not seen are eternal."

Psalm 103:3
"Who forgiveth all thine iniquities; who healeth all thy diseases."

Matthew 4:23
"And Jesus went about all Galilee, teaching in their synagogues, and preaching the gospel of the kingdom, and healing all manner of sickness and all manner of disease among the people."

I Peter 2:24
"Who his own self bare our sins in his own body on the tree, that we, being dead to sins, should live unto righteousness: by whose stripes ye were healed."

Isaiah 53:4-5
"Surely he hath borne our griefs, and carried our sorrows: yet we did esteem him stricken, smitten of God and afflicted. But he was wounded for our transgressions, he was bruised for our iniquities: the chastisement of our peace was upon him; and with his stripes we are healed."

Proverbs 23:7
"For as he thinketh in his heart, so is he: Eat and drink, saith he to thee; but his heart is not with thee."

Philippians 4:8
"Finally brethren, whatsoever things are true, whatsoever things are honest, whatsoever things are just, whatsoever things are pure, whatsoever things are lovely, whatsoever things are of good report; if there be any virtue, and if there be any praise, think on these things."

Proverbs 17:22
"A merry heart doeth good like a medicine: but a broken spirit drieth the bones."

Proverbs 3:8
"It shall be health to thy navel, and marrow to thy bones."

Health & Wellness

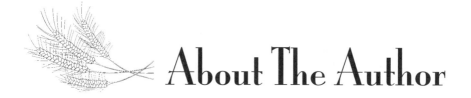# About The Author

Dr. Calvin Ellison is an anointed teacher who flows under an apostolic and prophetic mantle. He is the Pastor of Oasis of Hope Church in Farmville, North Carolina. He has a mandate to the nations of the world and has thus traveled to Haiti, England, Bulgaria and various countries in Africa.

Dr. Calvin Ellison holds a PhD of Ministry from Central Christian University. He is also a Naturopathic Doctor who earned his degree from Trinity College of Natural Health. He is a certified Nutritional Consultant with AANC (American Association of Nutritional Consultants). He is also the Founder of Success Dynamics Community Development Corporation which houses such programs as: East Coast Restorative Academy, Women's Empowerment Network, Mentors in Action and The Community Empowerment Network (a collaboration of churches focused on empowering the community – economically, educationally and health wise). Dr. Calvin Ellison is also the Vice Chairman for the Mid-Eastern North Carolina Community Development Corporation and the spokesman for Circle of Faith, Inc. He is currently serving on the Cultural Competency Committee for the state of North Carolina's Mental Health Reform and served on the Board of the Chamber of Commerce in Farmville, North Carolina.

Dr. Ellison is married to Dr. Judy Ellison who is the co-Pastor of Oasis of Hope Church. Called by God since 1985, they have ministered to thousands about marriage--using seminars, banquets, retreats, television and radio--teaching and instructing them how to become "Heirs Together."

Dr. Calvin and Judy Ellison are the authors of several quote books which include: Wisdom Keys for Great Marriages, Wisdom Gems for Singles, Wisdom Nuggets for Wellness, Ten Nutritional Keys for Children, Proverbs for Women in Ministry, and Health & Wellness School Workbooks.

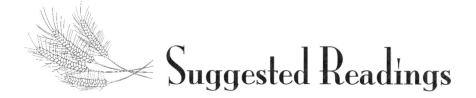

Suggested Readings

Natural Cures They Don't Want You to Know About
Kevin Trudeau
Alliance Publishing

Never Be Sick Again
Raymond Francis, M.Sc
HCI

The Truth about the Drug Companies
Marcia Angell, M.D.
Random House Trade Paperbacks

How to Feel Great All the Time
Valerie Saxion, N.D.
Bronze Bow Publishing

Walking in Divine Health
Don Colbert, M.D.
Siloam Press

Colon Health
Dr. Norman Walker
Norwalk Press

Go Natural
Mark & Patti Virkler
Destiny Image Publishers

Other Books & Tapes by Dr. Ellison

Health & Wellness Manuals (Vol. 1 & 2)

Wisdom Keys for Great Marriages (quote book)

Wisdom Gems for Singles (quote book)

Wisdom Nuggets for Wellness (quote book)

For seminars or health & wellness school workshops contact:

Dr. Calvin Ellison
Vibrant Life Health Seminars
P.O. Box 214
Farmville, NC 27828

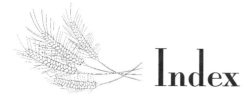

Index

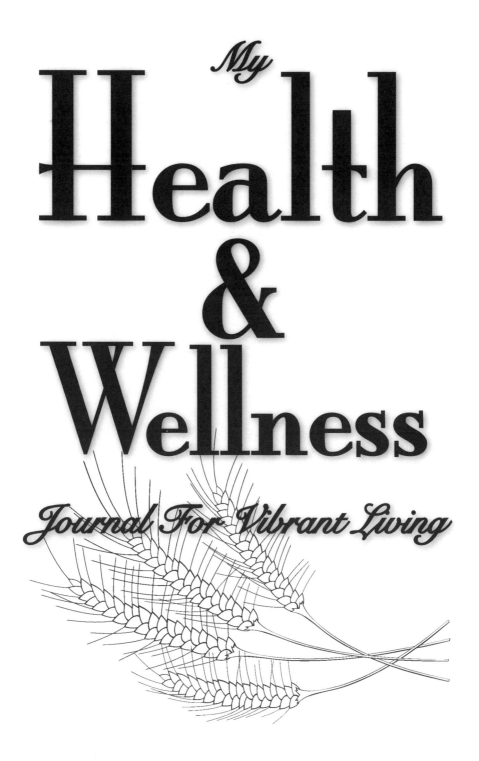

My

Health
&
Wellness

Journal For Vibrant Living

"And said, If thou wilt diligently hearken to the voice of the LORD thy God, and wilt do that which is right in his sight, and wilt give ear to his commandments, and keep all his statutes, I will put none of these diseases upon thee, which I have brought upon the Egyptians: for I am the LORD that healeth thee." Exodus 15:26

Journal

" He sent his word, and healed them, and delivered them from their destructions. " Psalm 107:20

"My son, attend to my words; incline thine ear unto my sayings. Let them not depart from thine eyes; keep them in the midst of thine heart. For they are life unto those that find them, and health to all their flesh. Keep thy heart with all diligence; for out of it are the issues of life."

Proverbs 4:20-23

" But he was wounded for our transgressions, he was bruised for our iniquities: the chastisement of our peace was upon him; and with his stripes we are healed. "

Isaiah 53:5

"And Jesus went about all Galilee, teaching in their
synagogues, and preaching the gospel of the kingdom,
and healing all manner of sickness and all manner of
disease among the people." Matthew 4:23

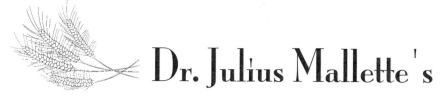

Dr. Julius Mallette's

Methods of Nutrition and Weight Management

Open a can of Whup Phat

© mallette 2006

Dr. Mallette's Steps to Happy Weight Loss and Maintenance

W -   walking, walnuts, water, working, waiting
H -   heaven, hope, happiness, humor
U -   understanding, U (you), umbrella, upset
P -   persistence, pleasure, power, pills- vitamin
PH F - forgiveness, fat-free, fun-meal, fiber
A -   accolades, apples, alright, ***ab-iso-belt*** patent pending
T -   tenacity, today , tomorrow, twice a day

I developed this weight loss technique after nearly 10 years of trying to maintain a healthy body weight and control adult onset diabetes (type II).

Success of the technique is based on the use of diet and exercise strategies that work for those of us that enjoy food and do not have a lot of time and money to spend at a gym.

The main diet strategy is to eat one main meal a day and small protein rich snacks at other times. The main meal must be before 7 pm or 4 hours before resting for the day. This allows for the full digestion of the meal. The snacks must include milk products if you are not allergic.

The main exercise strategy is to walk, walk, walk, walk and walk some more. At least 30 minutes a day preferably one hour a day. Using the ab-iso-belt will enable the wearer to perform iso metric abdominal exercise without trying.

W -   walking, walnuts, water,
       working, waiting

H -   heaven, hope,
       happiness, humor

U -   understanding, U (you),
       umbrella, upset

P -   persistence, pleasure,
       power, pills of vitamins only

PH F - forgiveness, fat-free,
       fun-meal, fiber

A -   accolades, apples,
       alright, ab-iso-belt

T -   tenacity, today ,
       tomorrow, twice-a-day

The
Ab-Iso-Belt

Patent Pending

Find out more about Dr. Julius Mallette's methods of nutrition and weight management. Go to --

www.whupphat.com